THE MANAGEMENT OF
ADVANCED PROSTATE CANCER

Dedicated to the memory of Freddy.
One learns from every patient.

The Management of Advanced Prostate Cancer

Malcolm J. Coptcoat
ChM, FRCS
Consultant Urologist
King's College Hospital
Denmark Hill
London SE5
UK

Blackwell
Science

© 1996 by
Blackwell Science Ltd
Editorial Offices:
Osney Mead, Oxford OX2 0EL
25 John Street, London WC1N 2BL
23 Ainslie Place, Edinburgh EH3 6AJ
238 Main Street, Cambridge
   Massachusetts 02142, USA
54 University Street, Carlton
   Victoria 3053, Australia

Other Editorial Offices:
Arnette Blackwell SA
   224, Boulevard Saint Germain
   75007 Paris, France

Blackwell Wissenschafts-Verlag GmbH
   Kurfürstendamm 57
   10707 Berlin, Germany

   Zehetnergasse 6
   A-1140 Wien,
   Austria

First published 1996
Reprinted 1997

Set by DP Photosetting, Aylesbury, Bucks
Printed and bound in Great Britain by
Hartnolls Ltd, Bodmin, Cornwall

The Blackwell Science logo is a trade mark of
Blackwell! Science Ltd, registered at the
United Kingdom Trade Marks Registry

DISTRIBUTORS

Marston Book Services Ltd
PO Box 269
Abingdon
Oxon OX14 4YN
(Orders: Tel: 01235 465500
          Fax: 01235 465555)
USA
Blackwell Science, Inc.
238 Main Street
Cambridge, MA 02142
(Orders: Tel: 800 215-1000
               617 876-7000
          Fax: 617 492-5263)
Canada
Copp Clark Professional
200 Adelaide Street, West, 3rd Floor
Toronto, Ontario M5H 1W7
(Orders: Tel: 416 597-1616
               800 815-9417
          Fax: 416 597-1617)
Australia
Blackwell Science Pty Ltd
54 University Street
Carlton, Victoria 3053
(Orders: Tel: 3 9347 0300
          Fax: 3 9347 5001)

A catalogue record for this title
is available from the British Library
ISBN 0–86542–929–4

Library of Congress
Cataloging-in-Publication Data

The management of advanced prostate
   cancer/Malcolm J. Coptcoat.
       p.   cm.
   Includes bibliographical references
   and index.
   ISBN 0–86542–929–4
   1. Prostate—Cancer. I. Title.
   [DNLM: 1. Prostatic Neoplasms–therapy.
   2. Prostatic Neoplasms–diagnosis.
   WJ 752 C785m 1996]
RC280.P7C68   1996
616.99'463–dc20
DNLM/DLC
for Library of Congress   95-40740
                                         CIP

Contents

Preface

Prostate cancer is now the most common neoplasm in men in the Western world and the second leading cause of cancer death after lung cancer. More than 90% of newly diagnosed patients referred to King's College Hospital in London present with locally advanced or metastatic prostate cancer, and this is one of the few hospitals in the UK which encourages screening of men over 60 years for prostate cancer, in the hope that localized disease can be caught early and treated. This is in contrast to the USA where the figure has been around 50%. But such clinical staging has been shown to be inaccurate and up to a further 50% of patients initially regarded as being suitable for radical surgery are found to have extracapsular extension and should have been reclassified as locally advanced. The sad conclusion is that the majority of prostate cancer patients in the West, at the present time, even with the sophistication of a sensitive tumour marker, are advanced and treatment is probably only palliative. The upbeat corollary is that such palliation can be life changing, long lasting and may yet provide the vital clue to enable us to one day cure not just those who may not have needed curing.

What are these treatment options? Many books on prostate cancer provide specialized accounts written by 'leaders in their field'. This book is different. Firstly, because it is problem-oriented and secondly, because it is a monologue that represents the continuity of thought of one leading hospital's urology department. It does not claim to be right, even less to be the definitive work. But it does contain plans, and their rationale, that we utilize on a daily basis for our patients. You are invited to read, accept or leave and possibly follow such plans, without the sometimes confusing presentation of opposite points of view. I have tried to summarize my strategy at the end of each chapter with 'Practice points'. The reader should begin to see how our ideas interlock and will find helpful advice for widely shared clinical problems.

ACKNOWLEDGEMENTS   I am grateful to Elizabeth, Marion and Heli for their help in preparing the manuscript. Whilst the references for this short book are both numerous and diverse, I must acknowledge the writing and influence of the late Geoffrey Chisholm CBE ChM FRCS.

Introduction

There are three main issues discussed in this book. The first is the need to consider the presentation of prostate cancer in the light of radical prostatectomy findings and the refinement of molecular staging. If advanced cancer is defined as that which has spread either locally or distantly, then sadly the vast majority of prostate cancer patients are presenting with advanced disease. This is despite the widespread use of the introduction of limited screening with the sensitive tumour marker in the form of prostatic specific antigen (PSA), and an increased awareness and education of patients.

Advanced prostate cancer, sadly shown by recently introduced molecular staging techniques to exist in more of our patients than previously thought, is unlikely to be cured by either surgery or radiotherapy. Treatment must be palliative until a combined strategy with a probable winning formula of surgical debulking, hormone manipulation, and chemotherapy is discovered. This is not for want of trying and the methods utilized are discussed in this book, and so the second issue is one of treatment and its timing. Delay in progression of disease and an increase in survival time are not unreasonable objectives whilst we await the ultimate cure. Early treatment of low volume disease by maximum androgen blockade seems to have provided this compromise but the evidence is not uniform. Given the diagnosis of malignant disease, the majority of patients wish for active treatment. This would be acceptable if it was not for the fact that some advanced prostate cancers are so slow growing that treatment is not required – at least for as long as expected survival is not altered by advances in health and health care in general – and that such hormonal treatment may have unpleasant side effects. The side effects of maximum androgen blockade have been reduced with the introduction of new anti-androgens, but the cornerstone of management in the absence of a definitive cure is data on quality of life issues. Controlled comparative trials using quality outcome measures are in progress and we eagerly await the results. Until then, much of our decision making will be based on a compromise between personal anecdotes, hand-me-down dogma, and hundreds of incompatible trials.

The third issue that is taken up in this book is the holistic approach to the patient's care. This does not mean the abandonment of science for the elusive herb: it is the recognition that the patient must be educated so that he can understand how to live, and sometimes die with his disease, but without anxiety. The terminal illness must be managed by an all-round palliative care team that involves hospital, hospice, and community personnel. Whilst we are still awaiting the ability to cure cancer, we can at least focus on the need to eradicate every cell of anxiety that may occur in our patients and their families lives whilst they have to live with the diagnosis of advanced prostate cancer.

Chapter 1
Natural History

Epidemiology

In Western men, cancer of the prostate is responsible for 20% of all malignancies and after cancer of the lung, is the second leading cause of cancer death (Table 1.1 & Fig. 1.1).

Table 1.1 Cancer deaths in males (1990).

	Death (%)
Melanoma of skin	3
Oral	4
Lung	25
Pancreas	3
Stomach	3
Colon and rectum	15
Prostate	20
Urinary	15
Leukaemia	7
All others	15

The geographical distribution in age adjusted mortality rates shows the highest values in Sweden, Switzerland and Norway, with the lowest in Taiwan, the Philippines and Japan (Fig. 1.2). Several studies have shown an increase in mortality rates for immigrants moving from a low incidence to a high incidence area; the implied environmental and dietary factors, rather than genetic, could account for such geographical differences, but differences in diagnostic effort and pathological interpretation cannot be discounted and remain the most likely reason for these discrepancies.

A consistent epidemiological finding is the high occurrence of the disease in black as compared to white American men; there is also a striking difference between the high incidence in black Americans and the low incidence in west Africans. Epidemiological studies of these two black populations have shown a significant positive association between prostatic carcinoma and sedentary occupation, sexual activity and venereal disease in

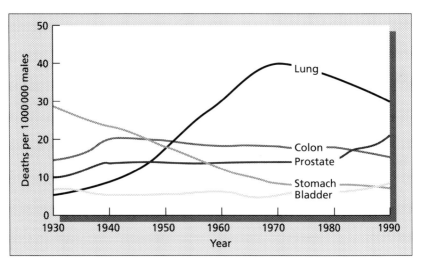

Fig. 1.1 Prostate cancer is the second most common cancer in males in the USA and Europe. It accounts for approximately 20% of all cancer deaths in males and this death rate has remained almost steady over the past 40 years (unlike that for lung cancer, which has increased and for stomach and colorectal cancer, which have decreased). (After Buck A.C. (1995) *Prostate Cancer. Questions & Answers.* Merit International, Hampshire.)

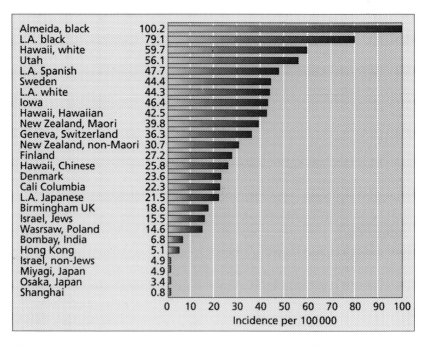

Fig. 1.2 Incidence of prostate cancer among various regions and ethnic groups based on autopsy findings. Some of these variations are enormous and must reflect different standards of reporting. (After Buck A.C. (1995) *Prostate Cancer. Questions & Answers.* Merit International, Hampshire.)

both groups, but apart from presenting at an early age in Americans and a later stage in Africans, there are no clear factors that account for the different incidences. Thus, while the differences between the American black and white male remain unexplained, they do suggest that there is a carcinogen more common to blacks in the USA.

An analogy between male prostate cancer and female cervical cancer has been made since both malignancies have a strong positive association with several criteria of sexual activity. The mortality rates for carcinoma of the prostate in the USA are strongly associated with marital status, being lower in single and higher in divorced men. There is now evidence of a relationship between sexual activity and venereal transmission in patients with prostatic cancer. Genital herpes virus (type II) found in the male urinary tract in the absence of overt disease has now been demonstrated in prostatic cells in patients with prostate cancer (Dmochowski & Horoszewicz 1976). An increase in antibody titre for both this virus and cytomegalovirus has been demonstrated in patients with carcinoma of the prostate, findings similar to those described in patients with cancer of the cervix. Several studies of malignant tissue have shown the presence of particles resembling C type RNA virus, and while these observations cannot be used to prove a cause or relationship, they indicate the need for further study.

The relationship between prostate cancer and social class is still debatable. Despite the problems in analysing and interpreting hospital records, a study has shown an increased incidence with a decreasing socioeconomic class. There was also an increased incidence in certain sections of social class one, e.g. doctors, an observation open to many interpretations (Hakky 1979).

Other clues have been sought from the known low mortality rate in Jewish men, and association persists with social class. A familiar incidence has been suggested by some American studies. There is inconsistent data associating incidents of men living in either cities or in the country. More definite associations have been reported with the rubber and cadmium industries. Just as benign prostatic hypoplasia has been linked with changes in serum hormones, so the development of malignancy has been seen as an extension of these changes. Several observations have suggested that both androgens and especially oestrogens may be involved. Patients with cirrhosis of the liver have less prostatic cancer than controls; prostate cancer is unknown in castrated men and both castration and oestrogen therapy have a palliative effect on advanced prostate cancer. Most comparisons between patients with cancer of the prostate and normal subjects have shown either very small or no significant differences in the testosterone and dihydroxytestosterone levels. This is not surprising considering the wide range of values reported in such studies. It is likely that the relationship between prostate tissue and serum hormone concentrations will be more relevant to carcinogenesis theories based on hormones.

Biological variation

In 1988, an estimated 90 000 cases were reported in the USA and some 26 000 of these died of their disease. At the same time, 14 000 cases were reported in the UK of which 4000 died of their disease. Murphy and colleagues (1982) reported that 25% of prostate cancers present as local disease, whilst Harbitz (1972) showed that 95% of prostate cancers are sub-clinical and microscopic.

Carcinoma of the prostate is common and its incidence increases progressively with age (Fig. 1.3). Approximately 25% of men in their sixth decade will have a focus of carcinoma or prostatic intra-epithelial neoplasia (PIN). In epidemiological surveys a large discrepancy is known to exist between incidence of the tumour and a death directly attributable

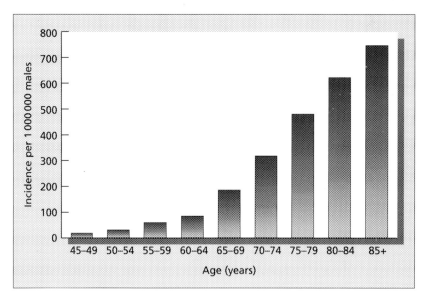

Fig. 1.3 Prostate cancer is virtually unknown in men aged below 45 years, but the incidence increases with age. Eighty-five per cent of prostate cancer patients are over 65 years. Although the peak age for new diagnosis is about 70 years, the age incidence continues to rise. This is because there are fewer men, at risk, due to death from other causes. Also the proportion of elderly men in the population is increasing. (After Buck A.C. (1995) *Prostate Cancer. Questions & Answers.* Merit International, Hampshire.)

to it. Many patients have up until now died within 5 to 10 years of the diagnosis from diseases other than prostate cancer. Although the implication is that most prostate cancer is therefore characterized by an indolent growth, it still ranks as the third commonest cause of cancer death in males in the USA and the UK, especially among those of Afro-Caribbean descent.

Although 20% of all men over 50 years old have cancer of the prostate at a microscopic level, only 5% of all men at a mean and median age of 65 years have a cancer greater than 1 cc in volume (Stamey *et al.* 1993). Depending on the patient's age and recognizing the slow doubling time of prostate cancer, it is therefore questionable whether prostate cancers less than 1 cc in volume require treatment.

Latent prostatic cancer

The frequent occurrence of latent carcinoma has been confirmed by many authorities, including Baron (1940). Our histological diagnosis is now much more refined and accurate, and Scardino & Wheeler (1988) have demonstrated that the autopsy prevalence of prostatic adenocarcinoma reaches 30% in the seventh decade, 40% in the eighth decade and 50% in the ninth decade. Interestingly, incidental cancers in other organs at autopsy are a relatively rare finding at any age. Hence, for the prostate, a unique dichotomy exists between the magnitude of the reservoir of malignancy in the population and the rate of emergence of clinically aggressive disease. Scardino has calculated, using a 30% overall prevalence figure, that only 1.05% of the total population reservoir of cancer reaches clinical diagnosis in any year and the annual mortality rate is only 0.31% of the total prevalence of histological cancer. It was Franks (1954) who proposed that two distinct species of carcinoma occur in the prostate; the latent variety accounts for the high overall prevalence of the cancer, and is the biological form incapable of even acquiring malignant behavioural features. This concept of latency as originally proposed is untenable if it is not correlated with at least an histological grade: the carcinomas are not necessarily of low grade, although the majority are. This view has been further supported by the observation that the prevalence of incidental cancer is high in countries where the incidence of clinical cancer is much lower than USA levels. These latent cancers possibly represent a completely different biological variation but there is epidemiological evidence that they can be 'switched on'. This is seen in the first generation Asian immigrants into Western society.

The mean prostatic specific antigen (PSA) doubling time in untreated patients is measured in years. In contrast, the PSA doubling time is measured in only a few months in those patients who have failed radical surgery or radiotherapy, which begs the question that intervention may actually be adversely affecting the natural history of the tumour.

Prostate cancer usually presents in an advanced stage often with metastases. Usually patients seek medical advice because of local symptoms of prostatism, but occasionally symptoms from metastases for example hip or low back pain maybe the presenting complaint. Occasionally one comes across an occult or silent metastasizing carcinoma and these neoplasms do not differ morphologically or histologically from other prostate carcinomas. The large discrepancy in the number of recorded deaths and incidence of prostate cancer is due to the large number of latent cancers. Although some studies have defined a latent prostatic cancer found at autopsy, it is not unreasonable to assume that these cancers are behaving in a completely different way. They account for the majority of prostate cancers diagnosed in Far Eastern countries where the death rate attributable to prostate cancer is even lower than that found in Western society.

Metastatic potential

Histological perivascular and perineural invasion and its close correlation with progressive disease, is a microscopic development of the potential for angiogenesis in an individual tumour. In some patients, metastases develop many years after the removal of the primary tumour and apparent cure. Several non-mutually exclusive hypotheses have been proposed to explain the dormancy of metastases. The sudden conversion of quiescent actively divided cells could occur by a change in cell cycle with progression from a G0 to a G1 phase. The factor that would initiate this conversion is unknown. Alternatively, the size of tumour metastases may be kept in check by host specific and non-specific immunity so that a change in antigenicity or suppression of host immunity, may tip the balance in favour of the tumour cells. Trauma of normal tissues is usually followed by inflammation and repair, which depends on production of organ specific growth factors. These factors can also stimulate the proliferation of tumour cells, possessing the appropriate receptors. Whether trauma also produces a switch to the angiogenic phenotype in tumour cells, is unclear. In any case, an increased understanding of the process of angiogenesis, which is directly related to the development of metastases, has led to the recent hypothesis that the end of tumour dormancy may be explained by a sudden conversion of a tumour to the angiogenic phenotype. This may occur by an increase in angiogenesis stimulators, a decrease in angiogenesis inhibitors, or a combination of the two. Elucidation of the factors governing tumour angiogenesis may help to sort out this phenomenon.

The major barriers to the treatment of metastases are the biological heterogeneity of cancer cells, and the rapid emergence of tumour cells with resistance to most conventional anti-cancer agents, which in the case of prostate cancer, is a relative form of androgen independence. Inhibition of angiogenesis however provides a novel and more general approach for treating metastases by manipulation of the host micro-environment. Endothelial cells in tumour blood vessels divide rapidly, whereas those in normal tissues do not. The division of endothelial cells is induced by a variety of mitogens, termed angiogenic factors. Systemic administration of antibodies to basic fibroblast growth factor (bFGF) (Hori 1991), vascular endothelial growth factor (Kim 1993), or angiogenin (Olson 1994), has been shown to inhibit the *in vivo* (but not *in vitro*) growth of tumour cells, suggesting tumour growth may be inhibited indirectly by inhibiting angiogenesis. Treating neoplasms by targeting both the tumour cells (hormone therapy and chemotherapy) and the organ environment (angiogenesis inhibitor), has been shown to reduce additive or synergistic therapeutic effects in mice bearing the 3LL tumour (Teicher 1994). This conclusion is contrary to the once accepted idea that metastases represents the ultimate expression of cellular anarchy. The view that cancer metastases is selective implies that understanding the mechanisms that regulate the process may lead to better therapeutic intervention.

Cancer volume

A lot still remains unresolved regarding the natural history of adenocarcinoma of the prostate, but the weight of evidence indicates that this unpredictable label is not justified. Accurate knowledge of prostate cancer volume and histological grade can be highly predictive of its biological behaviour (McNeal *et al.* 1990). Prostatic adenocarcinoma is probably a single biological entity with a very high rate of malignant transformation, but a very slow and constant mass doubling time and a very slow biological progression rate; this is linked to cumulative cell division and hence to tumour volume (Fig. 1.4). The exception to this, as is the case with poorly differentiated tumours which can behave very virulently and can disseminate widely to soft tissues, proves the truth of this generality.

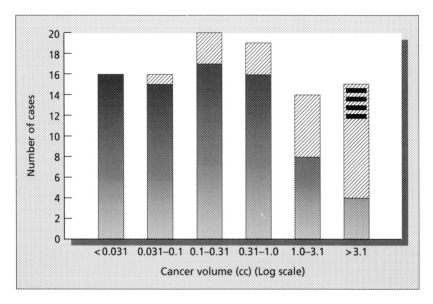

Fig. 1.4 Volume distribution of prostate cancer in 100 autopsies grouped into six consecutive, logarithmically equal volume intervals. Cases with Gleason grade 4 and/or 5 elements are indicated by hatched areas. Cases with distant metastases are indicated by horizontal bars. (After Stamey T.A., McNeal J. In: Campbells, *Urology*, p. 1162. WB Saunders, Philadelphia.)

Prostatic intra-epithelial neoplasia (PIN)

The term 'PIN' (prostatic intra-epithelial neoplasia) was proposed as a substitute for dysplasia. Evidence suggests that PIN is an early stage in the development of some prostatic carcinomas but the frequency with which this occurs and the interval between the two are unknown. It represents a carcinoma *in situ* but its behaviour is unpredictable and in many cases the disease does not progress. Its presence accounts for the previously reported high incidence of cancer in the normal population.

PIN is seen in over 80% of prostate specimens or biopsies associated with carcinoma but occurs in only 40% of prostates associated with hyperplasia in patients below the age of 60. In contrast, in those patients over 60 its association with carcinoma is similar but begins to appear in a much higher percentage in prostates with hyperplasia. The invasive carcinoma when present maybe adjacent to the PIN or elsewhere in the prostate. Early invasive cancers are thought to occur at sites of glandular outpouching and basal cell disruption (Greene 1991). A model of prostatic carcinogenesis has been based on the morphological continuum of PIN and the multistep theory of transformation (Fig. 1.5a). Similarly, a model has

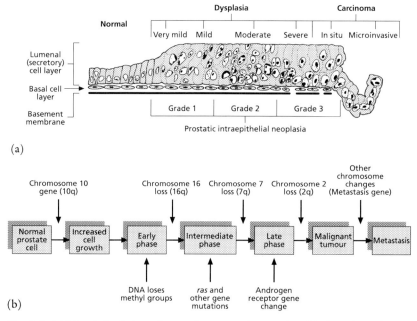

Fig. 1.5 (a) Morphological continuum from normal prostatic epithelium through increasing grades of PIN to early invasive carcinoma, according to the disease-continuum concept. Low grade PIN (grade 1) corresponds to very mild to mild dysplasia. High grade PIN (grades 2 and 3) correspond to moderate to severe dysplasia and carcinoma *in situ*. The precursor state ends when malignant cells invade the stroma; this invasion occurs where the basal cell layer is disrupted and the basement membrane fragmented. Notice that the dysplastic changes occur in the superficial (luminal) secretory cell layer, perhaps in response to luminal carcinogens. Disruption of the basal cell layer and basement membrane accompany the architectural and cytologic features of high grade PIN, and appear to be necessary pre-requisites for stromal invasion. (b) Proposed scheme of genetic events in prostatic carcinogenesis (Bostwick, 1992).

been proposed based on a series of putative genetic alterations involving tumour suppressor genes (chromosomes 7, 10, and 16) and oncogenes (Fig. 1.5b).

Genetic studies

Like breast cancer, the majority of prostate cancer is sporadic, but some familial clustering indicates that there is also a genetic susceptibility to the disease. It has recently been shown that about 10% of prostate cancer cases can be explained by the inheritance of genes given an autosomal dominant susceptibility. Again there is an age effect, with over 40% of cases diagnosed before the age of 55 being genetic. Male carriers of the susceptibility genes have a greater than 80% risk of disease by the age of 85, as opposed to a less than 5% risk for non-carriers. Additionally, families in Iceland with an inherited susceptibility to breast cancer, also showed increased frequencies of prostate cancer. If the familial prostate cancer gene is a tumour suppressor, its genomic location may be indicated by LOH studies on prostate tumours. LOH studies have found losses of chromosomes 7, 8p, 10q, 11p, and 16q. The 8p locus is additionally the fourth most frequent loss in CRC after chromosomes 18 (DCC), 5q (APC), and 17p (TP53). Chromosome 16q is the most frequent site of loss in breast cancer, indicating that these tumour suppressor genes may be involved in diverse tumour types. Once the chromosome 8p (CRC) and the 16q breast cancer tumour suppressor genes have been identified, it will be interesting to see if they are indeed mutated in prostate tumours, and if they are, whether there is any correlation with tumour progression.

The chromosome 10q loss seems to be specific to prostate cancer. This has been delineated by LOH studies to the 10q 23-qteR interval. Unfortunately, the amount of cytogenetic information on prostate cancer is relatively sparse when compared with that of common adenocarcinomas. This is mainly due to the frequent overgrowth of cultured slow growing cancer cells by normal cells. Nevertheless, cytogenetic analyses of prostate tumours have revealed frequent alterations involving the long arm of chromosome 10. Interestingly, chromosomal breaks seem to cluster at 10q 24, so this may be the site of the 10q prostate cancer tumour suppressor gene. Genetic markers in this region do also show linkage in prostate cancer families. Aprikian (1995) identified 329 patients with a positive family history out of a population of 2968 referred to a urology department with either a raised prostatic specific antigen (PSA) or an abnormal digital rectal examination (DRE). Prostatic cancer was diagnosed in 40% of those with a positive family history compared to 29% of those with no family history, producing an odds ratio of 1.7 for a positive family history and prostate cancer.

Chapter 2
Diagnosis and Staging

Historical perspective

It is interesting that until hyperplasia of the prostate began to be recognized as a separate entity in the early part of the 19th century, enlargement of the prostate was usually regarded as neoplastic. Two cases of undoubted carcinoma were described by Benjamin Brodie (1849). The first patient had lost weight and had suffered from sciatica; the prostate was found to be 'not much enlarged but of a stony hardness'. The second patient whose prostate was much enlarged and 'stony hard' developed excruciating pains in various parts of the body and became paraplegic – a syndrome which Brodie had observed in a patient dying of carcinoma of the breast with metastases in the spine. In the first half of the 19th century opinion as to the frequency of carcinoma of the prostate was reversed. Tanchou (1844) reviewed 1904 fatal cases of carcinoma in men and found only five reports of malignancy of the prostate. This low incidence parallels reported incidence in some under-developed countries in 1990 and may again reflect the lower mean age of survival in the general population. Prostate cancer is very much a problem of the developing world which cannot be ignored if we are to enjoy a longer life span. The typical osteoblastic metastases in bone were noted by Von Recklinghausen (1891) who based his report on five cases. Albarran & Halle (1900), in their study of the histology of enlarged prostates, found malignant changes in 14 of 100 glands. Between 1902 and 1907 H.H. Young found 21% of 318 cases of bladder neck obstruction to be associated with malignant changes, and in 1920 Freyer reported that 13.3% of his cases were carcinomatous. Recognition that prostate cancer was a much more common condition was therefore increasing. In 1935 Rich demonstrated carcinomatous changes in the prostate in 14% of all autopsies and in 28% of those aged over 70 years. Rich's figures seem to fit our experience in 1995 despite the claims in our undergraduate textbooks of vastly greater figures: inflated by the inclusion of what we now recognize as PIN. If the incidence of prostate cancer is lower than generally believed then the percentage of deaths, which we are sure of being attributable to it, is much larger and makes an interventional approach more reasonable.

Presentation of prostate cancer

The presentation of prostate cancer has changed dramatically because of the widespread use of prostatic specific antigen (PSA) as a tumour detection marker (see Prostatic specific antigen later). The increased number of patients presenting with asymptomatic localized disease because of such screening is encouraging and we may possibly expect to offer a cure for this group. However, an even greater number of patients are presenting with locally advanced disease with or without demonstrable metastases that have also been asymptomatic; some patients have only complained of minor prostatic symptoms. This larger group of patients presents a management dilemma unless one is convinced of the improved survival that prompt maximum androgen blockade would bring to these patients. Patients with prostate cancer have presented to us at King's College in the following groups:

1   localized disease (confirmed by radical surgical specimen assessment) (10%);

2   locally advanced disease with silent metastases (25%);

3   locally advanced disease with micro-metastases (including those understaged at radical surgery) (55%); or

4   locally advanced disease with symptomatic metastases (10%).

Molecular staging

Molecular staging has demonstrated that occult advanced prostate cancer often masquerades as local disease. As up to 50% of all patients with prostate cancer who have undergone radical prostatectomy are found to be under-staged subsequent to surgery, a more sensitive early staging modality has been required. A molecular assay that detects PSA – synthesizing cells in the peripheral circulation of patients with prostate cancer has been previously described. It utilized an enhanced reverse transcriptase-polymerase chain reaction (RT-PCR) assay specific for PSA mRNA. It was performed on RNA extracted from blood drawn from 94 patients before a radical pros-tatectomy. Surgical specimens were examined to determine the extent of tumour spread. The assay was compared with imaging modalities, digital rectal examination and serum PSA levels as predictors of the pathology and stage. In addition, patients were monitored post-operatively to determine any potential correlation between their pre-operative RT-PCR score and any subsequent tumour recurrence. Post-operative pathology revealed that 36 of the 94 patients had extra prostatic disease at the time of surgery and should therefore be reclassified as advanced tumours. Enhanced RT-PCR identified 26 of these patients from pre-operative blood specimens (72% sensitivity). The test was negative for 51 of the 58 patients with organ confined disease (88% specificity). An odds ratio analysis showed that no other pre-operative staging modality was related more strongly to either extra prostatic or organ confined disease. Follow-up PSA determinations revealed that the RT-PCR positive patients were at higher risk for a recurrence. This exciting work clearly confirms my impression that any impact that we will have on prostate cancer will come about with the use of systemic treatment. Although it would be interesting to receive the long term follow-up results from this study, there is already evidence that circulating PSA RNA reflects viable micro-metastases.

Incidental carcinoma

The finding of intra-prostatic focus of adenocarcinoma at autopsy which shows no evidence of spread is probably of little more than academic interest. Its frequency is directly proportional to the effort and enthusiasm which are taken by the individual pathologist in trying to locate such microscopic foci. However, the identification of a similar neoplastic focus within surgically resected tissue from a TURP has been more significant in that it immediately raises the controversial issue of possible further therapy and follow-up of that individual patient. Such carcinomatous foci are often small and isolated; the question that is often posed concerns the volume of prostatic tissue left given that the resected tissue would have come from the central and transitional zones and the majority of the residual tumour would be expected in the peripheral zone. The use of transrectal ultrasound (TRUS) scanning has been of great benefit in this area (see Transrectal ultrasound later). The frequency with which such a post-TURP diagnosis is made is also dependent upon the enthusiasm of the pathologist who may be very selective in his interest in the number of fragments presented to him.

Murphy and colleagues (1986) studied 386 consecutive prostatic resections from 383 patients with clinically benign glands; a carcinomatous focus was detected in 66 of those cases (17.2%). If histology from these cases had been limited to 12 g of randomly selected chips, only 90% of those incidental carcinomas would have been detected. In a similar study conducted by Moore's group (1986) all the resected prostatic chippings in 151 consecutive cases for benign prostatic hyperplasia were embedded for histology. Adenocarcinoma was diagnosed in 39 of these cases (25.8%). In two of their patients the number of fragments revealing carcinomas were

CHAPTER 2

smaller and counted for less than 1% of the total; this observation leads to the conclusion that to achieve a 95% level of accuracy, a minimum of 95% of the surgically resected tissue requires microscopic processing, which is not generally the procedure across the UK. There are two answers to this problem. The first is to be a little pragmatic: we conclude that those tumours missed truly *are* incidental and probably latent and their diagnosis would not affect the management of the patient. Our own records show that only 4% of these patients have died of their prostate cancer if the TURP was undertaken after their seventieth birthday. The second, and perhaps more reasonable and academic an answer, is to make greater use of fine needle aspiration biopsies and of selective sampling which sometimes shows that many of these tumours are locally advanced, but still do not always result in a cancer related death.

Prostatic specific antigen

Prostatic specific antigen (PSA) is transforming our management of prostate cancer. It is a highly sensitive tumour marker for:
1 tumour detection;
2 prognosis;
3 staging; and
4 follow-up.
PSA is one of the most abundant prostate-derived proteins in human seminal fluid. It is a 30 kDa glycoprotein whose primary structure manifests extensive structural similarity to that of the glandular kallikreins. The enzymatic activity for PSA has some features in common with chymotrypsin-like enzymes; its main role in the semen is one of the proteolysis of the sperm-entrapping gel formed in the ejaculate. This releases the progressively motile spermatoza. PSA occurs in human seminal fluid at levels of between 0.5 and 2 mg/ml. It is produced normally in prostate tissue; it is found in higher levels in infected and hyperplastic prostate tissue as well as cancer.

For screening purposes and tumour follow-up, PSA has proved to be a unique marker. However for prognostic purposes, it has not shown any superiority over grade and stage. Aggressive individual tumour cells seem to contain a lower PSA content, but as disease advances these will still produce a rise in serum levels. The level of serum PSA reflects the leakiness of the cancer cell membrane not the inherent PSA concentration in that cell. Because of this anomaly, other markers, such as tumour grade, seem to add more superior information.

It has been shown (Cooper *et al.* 1988) that a gram of benign, hyper-

14

plastic tissue produces more PSA and prostatic acid phosphatase (PAP) than the majority of prostate cancers. Normally there exists a blood/prostate barrier similar to the blood/brain barrier which prevents their widespread release into the circulation. However if that barrier is broken down by either, invasion of the capsule and extravesicular spaces by tumour cells; disruption of the stroma and connecting tissue elements of the gland during enormous hyperplasia; the presence of infection or by manipulation, these enzymes may be released into the circulation in significant concentrations. This occurs most significantly in the presence of metastatic disease. PSA is a more sensitive marker of capsular penetration than PAP (Siddall *et al.* 1986). Stamey and colleagues (1987) showed that tumours in lymph nodes tend to be associated with a slightly higher level of PSA than capsular penetration or seminal vesicle involvement. If the PSA is greater than 40 ng/ml, without any evidence of other metastatic disease, it is strongly suggestive that extensive lymph node involvement has already taken place. Other workers such as Freiha (1989) have suggested that the critical level of PSA in these cases is even lower and could probably be taken as 10 ng/ml.

Once the prostatic tumour has spread beyond the confines of the gland and metastasized distally as it usually does to bone, then occasionally very high levels of both PSA and PAP may appear. However it is possible for patients to have widespread evidence of metastatic disease with both PSA and PAP levels within the normal range; levels may then be a reflection of the differentiation of the gland.

Serum PSA is related to cancer grade. Patients with Gleason grade 4 and 5 (see The Gleason system later) have a markedly higher PSA value compared to those with lower grades. The more differentiated the tumour, the lower the tumour PSA content as measured by immuno-histochemistry. The mean serum PSA value in patients with tumours graded 3 or below is 10 ng/ml compared to 29 ng/ml in those with higher grades. Patients with PSA serum values of 50 ng/ml or above have an almost 100% chance of having a Gleason grade 4 or 5 cancer. A reasonable explanation for this could be an increased density of cancer cells in the tumour and an increased productive capacity, causing leakage of PSA into the blood.

A proportion of PSA created in patients with carcinoma of the prostate occurs in the serum in complex with antichymotrypsin (ACT); this occurs in a higher proportion than in patients with benign prostatic hyperplasia (BPH): 90% versus 70% respectively (Christensson *et al.* 1993). This has further enhanced the sensitivity of PSA as a tumour marker. The molecular basis for the varying degree of complex formation between PSA and ACT in prostate cancer as compared with BPH is under further investigation, but the crucial observation may be that the PSA-containing prostate epithelium also produces ACT. This in turn may explain the haemolytic problems sometimes encountered during surgery of patients with advanced prostate cancer, even in the presence of supposedly normal bleeding and clotting parameters, because of the action of released *uncomplexed* PSA.

PSA changes in advanced prostate cancer

PSA has proved to be an extremely important marker in patients with prostate cancer. It has assumed a role in early detection, staging and identification of residual disease after radical prostatectomy or radiation therapy. In addition, the overwhelming majority of patients with metastatic carcinoma or locally advanced prostate cancer have an abnormal serum level of PSA. Less certain however are changes in PSA which occur with hormonal therapy and more importantly whether these changes can be used to predict the outcome in individual patients. PSA changes with endocrine therapy should reflect an impact of the therapy upon the disease process, but they may also be an indication of the androgen dependence of the mechanism of PSA production, independent of tumour response.

In general, studies have shown that normalization of PSA after approximately 3 months of endocrine therapy is a better predictive parameter for the duration of response than either percentage decrease or normalization at any other time point. This phenomenon is also seen in those studies comparing maximal androgen blockade (MAB) with monotherapy, and reinforce the concept of MAB for the routine management of advanced prostate cancer. These findings also raise the question of whether a more effective adjuvant therapy is required in those patients whose PSA fails to normalize after 3 months of endocrine treatment.

Serum PSA as a predictor of skeletal metastasis

The serum PSA concentration can reliably predict the absence of skeletal metastasis in patients with newly diagnosed untreated prostate cancer (Chybowski *et al.* 1991). In this study of 521 patients, the serum PSA was the best overall predictor of positive radionuclide bone scan findings. A staging radionuclide bone scan is not necessary for patients with newly diagnosed, untreated prostate cancer who have no skeletal symptoms and a serum PSA concentration less than or equal to 10 mg/ml.

Serum PSA, when combined with tumour grade and local clinical stage, can reliably predict on an individual basis the absence of positive pelvic lymph nodes (Oesterling *et al.* 1993). The medical records of 1632 consecutive patients with clinically localized prostate cancer who underwent a bilateral pelvic lymphadenectomy were reviewed. The findings were correlated with the pre-operative serum PSA, local clinical stage based on rectal examination and the histological tumour grade as determined from the biopsy. Using logistic regression analysis, these investigators determined the appropriate combination of values for the three pre-operative variables that would yield a full speculative rate of less then 3% if these variables were used to predict pelvic lymph node status. Some significant results emerged. For example, a patient with a Gleason grade 3, clinical stage T2a prostate cancer and a serum PSA concentration of 8 ng/ml or less, did not need a staging bilateral pelvic lymphadenectomy. When these criteria are applied to patients with a clinical stage T1a to T2b prostate cancer, approximately 60% do not require staging bilateral lymphadenectomy. When all the patients in the investigation were considered, 26% met the criteria for avoiding a pelvic lymphadenectomy. These findings are most important for men being managed with perineal radical prostatectomy or undergoing definite radiation therapy.

Applied anatomy

The prostate is a gland with a branched structure (30–40 branches) embedded in fibro-muscular connective tissue. The relative proportions of glandular and connective tissue varies widely, but there is a constant division of the gland into four distinct zones (McNeal *et al.* 1988) that reveal a different incidence of cancer. Figure 2.1 shows a staging modality section of

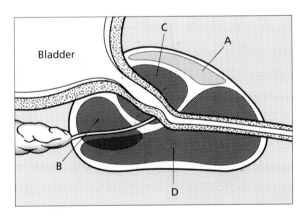

Fig. 2.1 The zonal anatomy of the prostate gland (see applied anatomy in text). The peripheral zone (D) gives rise to the majority (70%) of prostate cancers.

the prostate. The *anterior* zone (A) is purely fibro-muscular with no glandular elements. The *central* zone (B) contains the ejaculatory ducts; 8% of cancers occur in this zone. The *transitional* zone (C), composed of two lateral lobes, together with the periurethral glands, is the origin of the benign hyperplastic adenoma. It is also the origin of **25%** of prostate cancers and accounts for the majority of T0 lesions identified during a TURP for presumed benign hypoplasia. The *peripheral* zone (D) gives rise to **67%** of cancers and accounts for the value of the digital rectal examination (DRE) because of its proximity to the anterior wall of the rectum.

Imaging of advanced prostate cancer

Computed tomography and magnetic resonance imaging

Most computed tomography (CT) and magnetic resonance imaging (MRI) scans are ordered with the mistaken idea that they will clearly identify either intra- or extra-prostatic capsular spread and thus add useful information. Capsular penetration into the peri-prostatic fat and into the seminal vesicles is a microscopic phenomenon that is far from the resolving power of even a rectal coil MRI, unless exceedingly gross disease is present which should be detectable on rectal examination or indicated by the level of serum PSA (Fig. 2.2). TRUS, when combined with systematic biopsies, yields much better information than can ever be obtained with MRI or CT. Even so, TRUS is not a very sensitive imaging modality for detecting peri-prostatic or seminal vesicle invasion at the microscopic level.

If one follows the adage that an investigation is only warranted if the answer may change the course of management for an individual patient, then there is very little need for either MRI or CT of the pelvis in advanced prostate cancer except in the planning of radiotherapy. The presence of nodes will not alter the course of treatment. The presence of hydrone-phrosis or bone metastases may change the course of management but these can be much more easily identified with an *isotope bone scan* and *abdominal ultrasound* respectively.

The role of CT of the upper urinary tract is firmly established but MRI has become the first choice investigation for the assessment of locally advanced prostate cancer and the definition of spinal metastases. CT will only show gross pelvic lymphadenopathy. A pelvic (iliac and obturator node

Fig. 2.2 This transrectal ultrasound shows extracapsular spread (T3) of what had seemed at DRE to be a small nodule.

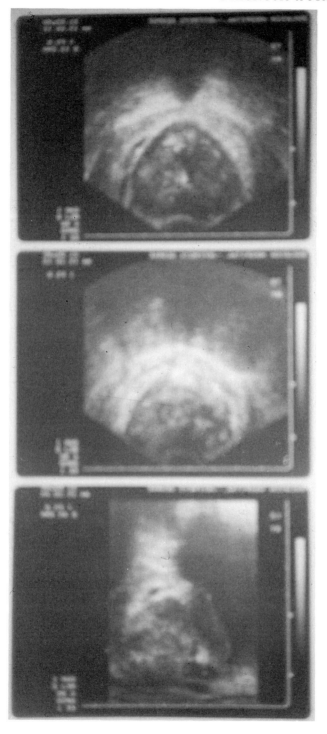

sampling) lymphadenectomy is required to detect micro-metastases, but this offers no extra information to manage a patient with advanced prostate cancer and is reserved in a laproscopic form for the confirmation of localized disease. We would use routine abdominal ultrasound scanning to confirm the diagnosis of a hydronephrosis that may be suggested by slow release of isotope from the kidney on a bone scan. Identification of the level of obstruction does then require the use of CT. It is rare for the level of obstruction to be in the mid or upper ureter in cases of prostate cancer, but paraaortic lymphadenopathy as a cause of ureteric obstruction does occur in up to 5% of patients and is best shown on CT. The more common site of obstruction is in the pelvis from locally advanced disease and this can be equally well demonstrated on both CT and MRI.

More space will be given to MRI in this book because of its emerging impact in the diagnosis of quiescent spinal metastases and any possible local complications that they may produce. MRI appears to be a safe technique and no ionizing radiation is required for the examination. It is not necessary to use iodonated contrast materials in MRI to achieve adequate contrast for purposes of diagnosis. Thus examinations may usually be performed in patients with marginal renal function. One must remember however that metal objects severely distract and distort the imaging process and any patients with a prosthesis should not be submitted to MRI. Even a patient with a small piece of residual shrapnel behind an eye is at risk when surrounded by the large magnetic field.

Nuclei that possess an odd number of either protons or neutrons demonstrate a property called spin. Nuclei with spin can produce a small magnetic field. These nuclei can be considered as tiny bar magnets whose lines of force show a definite magnitude and direction. In MRI the most important nucleus is the hydrogen nucleus because of its great abundance in biological tissues. In the absence of an externally applied magnetic field, these magnetically sensitive nuclei have a random orientation and there is no net magnetization in the body. When an external magnetic field is applied to a group of randomly orientated nuclei, they tend to align themselves along the direction of the applied magnetic field. Those aligning in the direction of the applied magnetic field tend to be more stable than those orientated in the opposite direction of the applied magnetic field. Once subject to the external magnetic field, the hydrogen nuclei exhibit a complex motion that is termed precession. Precession is the spinning and wobbling motion resembling that of a spinning toy top. The precessional frequency of the nuclei is in the radio frequency (RF) range. If an RF pulse is applied for a sufficient duration, the net magnetization may be deflected (tipped) at 90°

or even 180°. Immediately after the RF excitation, the excited spins are temporarily in phase and nuclei are precessing in synchrony. The return to the equilibrium state after the excitation pulse ceases is termed magnetic relaxation. Two exponential time constants described the return to the baseline equilibrium state; the T2 relaxation time, otherwise known as the spin or transverse relaxation time, and the T1 relaxation time, which is the exponential time constant that describes the regrowth of the longitudinal component of the magnetization after excitation.

The prostate gland is best seen on T2 weighted images when considerable intra-prostatic morphologic detail can be identified. Endorectal surface coil imaging has provided a major step forward in prostatic MRI, especially with regard to staging carcinoma of the prostate (Schnall 1991) but we have not found this to have had any major impact on management decisions and it is not part of our working routine. The neurovascular bundle is easily identified on axial views surrounding the prostate at the 5 and 7 o'clock positions, especially with surface coil images. The axial plane clearly demonstrates the zonal architecture of the prostate and also serves to identify the relations of the gland to surrounding fat and muscle. The relations of the prostate and the bladder, and extension of prostatic tumours into the bladder are best demonstrated on the sagittal images.

Transrectal ultrasound (TRUS)

Prostate cancer is hypoechoic but the degree of hypoechogenicity is variable and dependent upon the amount of solid tumour per unit area. Only macroscopic cancer can be detected on TRUS. A solid tumour can be anechoic, while an infiltrating tumour with equal or greater amounts of interposed normal glandular acini may be only slightly hypoechoic or nearly isoechoic. There is no hyperechoic cancer. Hyperechoic foci can be present in a cancer due to enveloped corpora amylacea and dystrophic calcification in necrotic tumour tissue, the actual hypoechoic background being overlooked due to focus on the more prominent bright echoes. Such cancers are usually identified as cribiform adenocarcinoma, the only form of adenocarcinoma having a distinctive differential pattern.

Concomitant new biopsy techniques have evolved along with improvements made in ultrasound imaging. The sensitive 7 MHz probes now facilitate a biopsy via the transrectal route (with antibiotic cover) whilst availability of an automatic biopsy device utilizing an 18 gauge Biopty needle has also improved the accurate placement of the biopsy needle. The transrectal route for prostate biopsy has certain advantages over the transperineal route because it is highly accurate for sampling lesions of approximately 1 cm in dimension, it is easily, quickly and safely performed, it is relatively painless, and does not require analgesia or sedation. Because of the possibility of infection, all patients should be prophylactically treated with an antibiotic. This can take the form of oral Norfloxacin taken 1 hour before the biopsy, or an intravenous injection of Gentamicin given just prior to the biopsy. It is sometimes difficult to obtain a biopsy by the transrectal route when a patient is either extremely anxious or there are associated local problems such as haemorrhoids which can produce quite severe pain on introduction of a probe. In these cases, it is better to carry out the biopsy under general anaesthesia because even a transperineal biopsy will require analgesia sedation and cannot be accurately guided without the use of TRUS.

The introduction of TRUS especially TRUS-guided biopsies of hypoechoic areas as opposed to blind finger-guided biopsies, has clearly increased the detection rate of prostate cancer in screening populations. Cooner and colleagues (1990) have published studies utilizing digital rectal examination (DRE), PSA testing and TRUS in 2648 between 50 and 89 years old who were referred to their urological practice. It is important to recognize from their data that the non-specificity of hypoechoic areas is in the peripheral and central zones of the prostate. If DRE was positive, 2.5 patients with hypoechoic areas needed biopsy for every cancer detected (732/288). If DRE was negative, 5.3 hypoechoic areas needed biopsy for every cancer discovered (504/95). Overall, regardless of DRE findings, 3.2 patients must undergo a biopsy because of hypoechoic areas for every patient proved to have cancer. Hypoechoic lesions in the peripheral and central zones of the prostate are not specific with cancer. As the average prostate extends for only 4 cm in the cephalocaudal direction, it is recommended that six systematic biopsy specimens taken under TRUS guidance are the best way to diagnose prostate cancer, when no visual abnormality exists but suspicion is provided by a raised PSA.

The role of TRUS in the management of prostate cancer should focus on the evaluation of a patient without demonstrable metastases, including molecular staging when possible, for curative treatment. TRUS is not needed for a clinically obvious advanced cancer, unless an unguided biopsy is negative. Evaluation of a patient for radical surgery or radiotherapy cannot be just dependent on the echo characteristics of the capsule. There have been 28% false negatives in our own series. This could possibly have been reduced by accurate capsule and peri-prostatic staging biopsies (Ravery 1994), but these advanced techniques are not yet widely practiced. However it is mandatory to at least perform a staging biopsy of the contralateral lobe, seminal vesicles and apex. It is only through meticulous staging biopsies that we will reduce the embarrassingly large number of patients who are understaged and undergo unnecessary radical treatment. At present it would not be unreasonable to recommend radical radiotherapy as the best alternative because it does least unnecessary harm. But this is an historical reflection. Improvements in staging may allow us to make a reasonable management plan that includes observation for the well differ-entiated and indolent tumour, surgery for the confirmed localized tumour in a younger man (< 72 years), radiotherapy for localized disease with either a high PSA suspicious TRUS findings, especially in an older patient and the informed option of MAB for those with proven advanced prostate cancer. We have not found that the routine use of either pelvic CT or rectal coil MRI has had a significant impact on this decision making process. Spinal MRI has a vital role in cases of suspected spinal cord compression and abdominal CT has a role in the assessment of a patient with suspected obstructive nephropathy secondary to advanced prostate cancer.

The radionuclear bone scan

Prostate cancer most commonly metastasizes to bone (Fig. 2.3). The infamous valveless veins of Batson are considered now by only the most naive to play a role in the spread of this cancer to the often affected spine and pelvis. Micrometastases are uniformly distributed in the vascular and lymphatic circulation. The establishment of a viable metastasis is more to do with the 'fertile soil' than the source of the 'seed'. The radionuclear bone scan using gamma camera images following an intravenous injection of a technitium salt can identify a potential bone metastasis long before it becomes apparent on a plain X-ray.

Simple technetium salts do not localize in the skeleton, but complexes or chelates of technetium with a number of phosphorous containing com-pounds do concentrate in bone. Some of these phosphonates can be used for therapeutic purposes. The basic mechanism underlying the concentration of the phosphonates in bone are incompletely understood, but there is strong evidence that they are bound to collagen and not bone mineral, as one might have expected. Blood supply is an important factor and calcium content is not. Hyperaemia is associated with a reduced calcium content, but an increased uptake of scintigraphic agents. The majority of abnormalities on a skeletal technetium-99 labelled bone scan appear as areas of increased uptake. However, some lesions present as photon deficient areas. Photon rich lesions are those in which osteoblastic activity is present, whilst

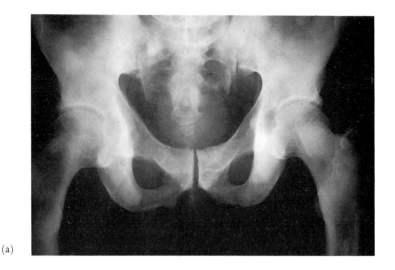

(a)

(b)

Fig. 2.3 (a) Skeletal metastases from prostatic carcinoma. Typical appearance of prostatic carcinoma. Typical appearance of prostatic bone metastases. Multiple sclerotic lesions are seen in the pelvis, sacrum, lumbar spine, and upper femora. Careful inspection also reveals a few small suggestive lytic lesions. (b) Isotope bone scan showing multiple metastases in the spine, pelvis and ribs.

osteoblastic activity is almost or totally absent in photon deficient abnormalities. Skeletal scintigraphy indicates the response of the normal tissue to the presence of a pathological process such as neoplasia or infection and is not a direct indicator of the pathological process itself. This is an important concept because it explains why bone scans cannot be used to accurately monitor progress of disease. A particular form of management such as radiotherapy or hormone treatment may produce a negative scan without destruction of the metastatic deposit. In these cases, a T2 weighted

MRI scan may be more helpful. However, the bone scan remains the most sensitive diagnostic tool that we have to detect small bone metastases in untreated patients. False positive results can be produced by recent trauma, infection, inflammatory joint disease, and Paget's disease. These can usually be excluded on clinical grounds together with a plain X-ray. False negative bone scans in untreated patients are extremely rare. Lesions may occur anywhere in the skeleton, however peripheral lesions in the absence of deposits in the spine, pelvis and ribs are sufficiently rare for routine scanning of the limbs and skull and omitted if the axial skeleton appears normal. One problem that can sometimes arise when interpreting a bone scan image is the recognition of a superscan. This occurs when focal lesions are so extensive that they coalesce to produce a relatively diffuse image. A single plain X-ray of the pelvis will again clarify this issue, as this is always abnormal in such cases.

A review of the last 100 bone scans in our hospital has reinforced the concept that a bone scan is entirely unnecessary if a patient with prostate cancer has a PSA of below 10 ng/ml (Fig. 2.4). This is only true for an untreated patient because therapy, especially hormone treatment, may often lower the serum PSA to near normal levels, reflecting a decrease in

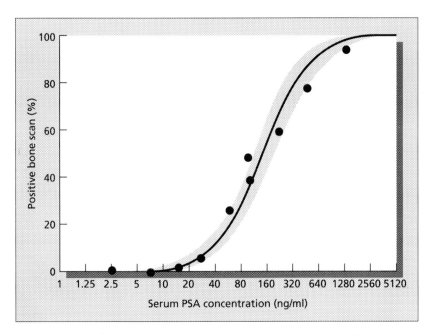

Fig. 2.4 Probability of a positive radionuclide bone scan as a function of the serum prostatic specific antigen (PSA) concentration. When the serum PSA is less than 10 ng/ml the probability of a positive bone scan approaches zero. (After Ekman P. *et al.* (1995) *J. Urol.* (*Scand.*), special issue on prostate cancer.)

PSA secretion by the cancer cells, but leaving the metastases still evident. Although for reasons given above, even the bone scan in these cases may be negative and a false hope of cure brought about that would be refuted with an MRI scan which would simply show the now dormant metastases. Our policy is to use a bone scan in the preliminary work-up of a patient with prostate cancer when the PSA is greater than 10 ng/ml. The use of bone scans in the follow up of treated patients needs to be reasonably rationed to those in whom a change of management might result. MRI has a more vital role as a sensitive diagnostic indicator of spinal metastases and possible soft tissue extension. Peripheral lesions are still best imaged by a bone scan.

Biopsy techniques

The diagnosis of prostatic cancer should always be confirmed if treatment of any kind is contemplated. The two main techniques are:
1   core biopsy with histopathological evaluation, and
2   aspiration biopsy with cytological evaluation.
Aspiration biopsies are now less popular because of the introduction of the Biopty instrument which consists of an 18 gauge needle core, 15 mm in length, which for most patients is less painful than aspiration biopsy. The Gleason grading system and its architectural classification also cannot be utilized in psychological grading and so very few centres are carrying out aspiration biopsies routinely.

The accuracy of a core biopsy can be significantly improved when the procedure is done under the guidance of TRUS and with a Biopty spring gun. There is still place for a finger-guided biopsy in an obvious T3 and T4 lesion where additional information from a TRUS is not needed.

Histopathology

The adenocarcinoma arising from the glandular elements of the prostate accounts for 98% of prostatic malignancy neoplasms. These often show a polymorphic appearance, varying from the small acini of a well differentiated tumour to the solid or trabeculated pattern of a poorly differentiated type. Other malignancies are rare in the prostate and include:
• transitional cell carcinoma (TCC) (1.5%) – the TCC is more often found to be locally invasive from the bladder;
• a rhabdomyosarcoma is found in children and young adults (0.3%); and
• a leiomyosarcoma in adults (0.25%).
Secondary tumours are vary rare.

The Gleason system

Prostatic cancer has a wide range of histological features and there is a close correlation between these features and the biological behaviour of the tumour. There are several systems of classification of the grade of the tumour but the most commonly used is that described by Gleason (1966).

Gleason's system is based on the analysis of various microscopic criteria of the tumour at low power magnification which are divided into five classical appearances, scored from 1 to 5. No tumour has a uniform appearance and the final score in this system takes into account this difference and is the summation of the two most differing appearances in terms of area (primary and secondary patterns). If a tumour contains smaller areas of other appearances they are not taken into account in the final histological grade, even if one of them corresponds to a more poorly differentiated pattern. Thus the histological grade is the sum of the two histological patterns defined, or twice the score of the single pattern detected. It is therefore scored from 2–10. In the Veterans Administration Co-operative Urological Research Group (VACURG), studies of the histological score at the initial biopsy was the most significant parameter for the assessment of the degree of malignancy of prostate cancer. The Gleason scoring system has come under criticism, particularly because of the poor reproducibility during repeated analyses by the same or by different pathologists. It is now being complemented by associated studies of DNA ploidy and other molecular markers, but will for the shorter term remain the backbone of our prostate cancer staging strategy.

Gleason's method only considers the degree of differentiation and the mode of growth of the tumour.

Grade 1 (Fig. 2.5) is very well differentiated adenocarcinoma. The tumour is composed of regular round or oval cells separated by a very fine stroma. These are arranged in very well defined clumps.

Grade 2 (Fig. 2.6) is a well differentiated adenocarcinoma where the tumour is composed of round or oval cells which are less uniform than in Grade 1 and separated by a slightly more abundant stroma. The clumps of tumour cells are also slightly less clearly defined.

Grade 3 (Fig. 2.7) is moderately differentiated adenocarcinoma where the tumour is composed of polymorphic differentiated glands, separated by abundant stroma and arranged in poorly defined clumps of invasive tumour

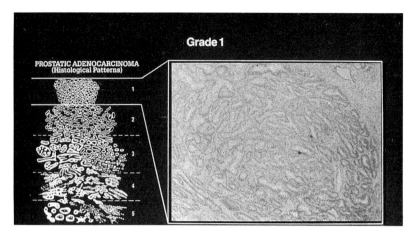

Fig. 2.5 Grade 1 is very well differentiated adenocarcinoma. The tumour is composed of regular round or oval cells separated by a very fine stroma. These are arranged in very well defined clumps.

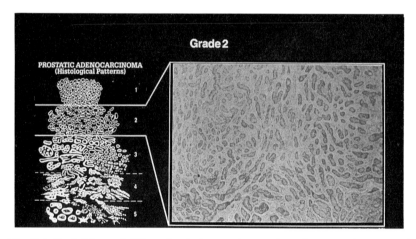

Fig. 2.6 Grade 2 is a well differentiated adenocarcinoma where the tumour is composed of round or oval cells which are less uniform than in Grade 1 and separated by a slightly more abundant stroma. The clumps of tumour cells are also slightly less clearly defined.

cells. Cribiform masses of sharp margins, which generally correspond to intra-duct tumour invasion are also included in this grade.

Grade 4 (Fig. 2.8) is poorly differentiated adenocarcinoma where the tumour is composed of poorly defined and poorly differentiated clumps containing poorly structured, fused glands. This grade also includes poorly defined polyadenomatous clumps and resemble pseudo-renal clear cell tumours.

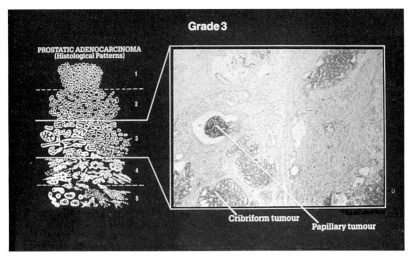

Fig. 2.7 Grade 3 is moderately differentiated adenocarcinoma where the tumour is composed of polymorphic differentiated glands, separated by abundant stroma and arranged in poorly defined clumps of invasive tumour cells. Cribiform masses with sharp margins, which generally correspond to intra-duct tumour invasion are also included in this grade.

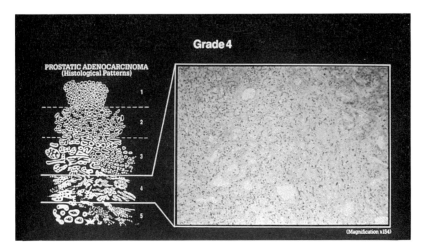

Fig. 2.8 Grade 4 is poorly differentiated adenocarcinoma where the tumour is composed of poorly differentiated clumps containing pooly structured, fused glands. This grade also includes poorly defined polyadenomatous clumps and resemble pseudo-renal cell tumours.

29

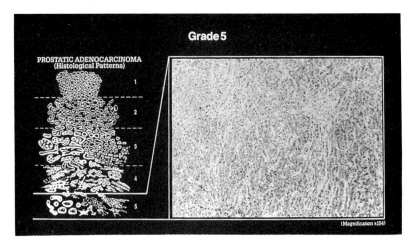

Fig. 2.9 Grade 5 is undifferentiated adenocarcinoma where there is minimal gland formation. The tumour is composed of bands, sheets or isolated cells with marked infiltration of the stroma. This grade includes tumours forming well defined compact masses with a necrotic centre which resemble mammary comedocarcinomas.

Grade 5 (Fig. 2.9) is undifferentiated adenocarcinoma where there is minimal gland formation. The tumour is composed of bands, sheets or isolated cells with marked infiltration of the stroma. This grade includes tumours forming well defined compact masses with a necrotic centre which resemble mammary comedocarcinomas.

TNM classification 1992

The TNM classification system describes the extent of a malignant disease in a patient thereby facilitating the categorization of that patient. It has a universal understanding and allows a better comparison of patients in diverse clinical trials. The 1992 revised classification was a consensus between the UICC and the American Joint Committee of Canar with support from the European Organization for Research and Treatment of Cancer (EORTC) and the Society of Urological Oncology. Future modifications will undoubtedly include parameters such as DNA ploidy, PSA and nuclear roundness factor thereby giving the system a more prognostic significance. At present this remains the language of choice; it should be applied meticulously if only to further endorse the correct treatment options that it does correspond to.

Incidental prostate cancer

Primary tumour (T)

TX   Primary tumour be assessed.
T0   No evidence of primary tumour.
T1   Clinically unapparent tumour, not palpable or visible by imaging.
T1a   Tumour an incidental histologic finding in 5% or less of tissue resected.
T1b   Tumour an incidental histologic finding in more than 5% of tissue resected.
T1c   Tumour identified by needle biopsy (e.g. because of elevated serum PSA).

Palpable or visible carcinoma confined to the prostate

T2   Tumour confined within the prostate

T2a   Tumour involves half a lobe or less.
T2b   Tumour involves more than half of a lobe but not both lobes.
T2c   Tumour involves both lobes.

Locally extensive prostate cancer

T3   Tumour extends through the prostate capsule

T3a   Unilateral extracapsular extension.
T3b   Bilateral extracapsular extension.
T3c   Tumour invades seminal vesicles.

Locally extensive tumour with fixation or invasion into neighbouring organs

T4   Tumour if fixed or invades adjacent structures other than seminal vesicles

T4a   Tumour invades bladder neck and/or external sphincter and/or rectum.
T4b   Tumour invades elevator muscles and/or is fixed to pelvic wall.

Regional lymph nodes (N)

NX   Regional lymph nodes cannot be assessed.

N0   No regional lymph node metastasis.

N1   Metastasis in a single regional lymph node, 2 cm or less in greatest dimension.

N2   Metastasis in a single regional lymph node, more than 2 cm but not more than 5 cm in greatest dimension; multiple regional lymph nodes, not more than 5 cm in greatest dimension.

N3   Metastasis in a regional lymph node, more than 5 cm in greatest dimension.

Metastatic disease

Distant metastases (M)

MX   Presence of distant metastasis cannot be assessed.

M0   No distant metastasis.

M1   Distant metastasis.

M1a   Non-regional lymph node(s).

M1b   Bone(s).

M1c   Other site(s).

Stage grouping 1992

Stage 0	T1a	N0	M0	G1
Stage I	T1a	N0	M0	G2, 3–4
	T1b	N0	M0	Any G
	T1c	N0	M0	Any G
	T1	N0	M0	Any G
Stage II	T2	N0	M0	Any G
Stage III	T3	N0	M0	Any G
Stage IV	T4	N0	M0	Any G
	Any T	N1, 2, 3	M0	Any G
	Any T	Any N	M1	Any G

Practice points

Routine investigations for a patient suspected as having prostate cancer because of an abnormal digital rectal examination (DRE) or raised prostatic specific antigen (PSA):

- Full blood count
- Serum PSA, creatinine and alkaline phosphatase
- Urine culture and microscopy
- Renal ultrasound (CT if hydronephrosis identified)
- Post micturition ultrasound (if flow rate over 100 ml)
- Transrectal ultrasound (TRUS) and guided biopsy (T0–T3)
- Simple outpatient random biopsy if T4

If biopsy positive:

Staging TRUS with biopsies if radial surgery considered

Bone scan (if PSA greater than 10 ng/ml)

Laparascopic pelvic lymphadenectomy (T0, T1, T2)

Plain X-ray if focal pain present

MRI of spine if bone scan positive in spine

Chapter 3
Hormonal Treatment

When the standard practice was to only treat prostate cancer patients with symptomatic metastases; when seemingly localized disease was tempered by the use of radiotherapy or endoscopic surgery; and when surgeons could sometimes claim to cure true localized disease, perhaps justifying the understaging that took place with a plea of mitigation on behalf of local control, it all seemed easy to follow. But there is now a general mistrust of these precepts and many urologists choose a variety of options still lacking a sensible basis.

The recent impact of molecular staging has left us with a further management dilemma. Given that over half of patients who have been traditionally labelled as having localized disease have really got either low volume locally advanced disease, or low volume disease with micro-metastases, then it is not enough to pat ourselves on the back and claim that we have at least avoided unnecessary surgery or radiotherapy in these patients. The impact to the patients' and families' combined psyche is almost incomprehensible when no treatment is offered. However, this should not make us run away from this responsibility if this is the correct choice for the patient. Early treatment of low volume disease does seem to lead to a prolonged survival, but it has not been conclusively shown that this is not simply a reflection of intervention at an earlier stage in the natural history of a patient's prostate cancer. We may only be affecting the lead time to progression rather than affecting the overall disease process.

Another situation which is just as psychologically demanding, if not to the patient then sometimes for the clinician, is when potentially curative treatment for presumed localized disease has failed. The management of a patient with residual or recurrent disease after attemptive curative radical surgery or radiotherapy remains a dilemma. One positive aspect is that we should find fewer patients in this situation in the future once a more discriminate free/total prostatic specific antigen (PSA) cut-off is universally employed and molecular staging using PCR-mRNA techniques have become widely used in the preliminary work-up of patients. But for the present time, and for at least 40% of patients who have undergone what they had hoped was radical treatment, we need a management plan. Residual or recurrent disease is most commonly identified by a positive or increasing

PSA result. A clinical presentation because of a previously silent metastases or obstructive or irritative systems for local regrowth is unusual in a world of PSA awareness. The ease of a biochemical test and its social significance is reinforced by dinner table conversations. Whilst the urological fraternity are debating the use of PSA for follow-up, and even screening, social pressures are slowly introducing the PSA test without any effect from us. 'What's your latest PSA result?' is at least as common a question as 'how's business?' amongst the middle class, middle aged, male dominated board rooms!

So one can be faced with an asymptomatic patient who perhaps has luckily retained not only his continence, but his potency. He is sitting opposite you with his wife. They have forgotten the 3 months of anxiety and convalescence from an operation that has faded from the memory 3 years previously. 'It was all so worth while. . . . Thank goodness the raised PSA was found at the annual medical. . . . Cancer surgery has become so clever. . . . We recommend you to all our friends'. Even with an ultra-sensitive PSA estimation, the previous follow-up results have been less than 0.01, less than 0.01 etc., but now, here it is: a serum PSA of 0.5 ng/ml; what does the clinician do? The consensus of opinion among urologists is divided. It is now clear that adjuvant radiotherapy for understaged cancers following surgery does not improve survival or delay progression to occult metastases (Hudson & Catalona 1990). This leaves us with the choice between doing nothing and starting early hormone treatment. Doing nothing is rarely accepted by patients in our Western culture, but must be considered in the light of our inability to actively define the patient's ulti-mate prognosis. Much will depend on the degree of differentiation or Gleason score of the initial tumour. The lead time to the development of metastases in patients with well or even sometimes moderately differ-entiated tumours can be up to 10 years. In the light of this natural history, it is probably unnecessarily unkind to submit such a patient to hormone manipulation without proven justification. Hormone treatment, even in the absence of identifiable side effects, often leaves the patient feeling slightly under par and this should only be tolerated together with the economic implications of sustained maintenance treatment if the patient can genu-inely feel that there is some ultimate benefit. Early treatment by hormone manipulation in the form of maximum androgen blockade (MAB), does have an enormous theoretical attraction because there can be no better defined low volume disease situation than this against which such systemic treatment may work. This argument is similar to that applied for MAB as a primary treatment option for clinically locally advanced disease and is dis-cussed later in this chapter.

The rationale for systemic treatment of prostate cancer should not always be applicable to every individual patient. Informed consent for a treatment regimen that should be indefinite is essential. Whilst it is my opinion that early intervention by MAB should be the first consideration in a patient with advanced prostate cancer, the possible outcome and side-effects should be understood by the patient and his family. It is quite reasonable to delay and possibly avoid systemic treatment of an elderly asymptomatic man, perhaps using a channel transurethral resection of the prostate (TURP) if local obstructive symptoms occur. But that patient has a right to know what the options were. He and his family will then begin to understand future management decisions, and the essential holistic approach based on a patient's trust will begin from the beginning.

Monotherapy

Bilateral orchidectomy

A bilateral orchidectomy has been the standard for hormone therapy since the report by Huggins and colleagues 1941. With the recognition of unexpected severe cardiovascular toxicity from 5 mg of Stilboestrol daily in the Veterans Administration Co-operative Urological Research Group (VACURG) studies, bilateral orchidectomy has been an attractive and important alternative to Stilboestrol therapy. It is the least expensive long-term therapy when compared with current non-Stilboestrol medical alternatives such as the luteinizing hormone-releasing hormone (LHRH) agonists and the non-steroidal anti-androgens. However, unlike medical treatment, a bilateral orchidectomy is not reversible and its main disadvantage is seen as psychological trauma to the patient with a generally permanent loss of libido and erectile impotence. It does however have the great advantage of complete therapeutic compliance and rapidly removes 95% of the most powerful circulating androgen, testosterone (Fig. 3.1). A bilateral orchidectomy can be performed safely and quickly with minimal morbidity on a day-case basis under local anaesthesia. If psychological resistance is expected, a subcapsular orchidectomy or even an artificial testicular implant can be performed, but this is an unusual request.

The majority of centres in the Western world have drifted away from this well proven method of hormone manipulation. This has in part been due to limited studies showing a patient preference for medical treatment (Parmar 1987; Chadwick 1991), but perhaps there has also been a laissez-faire effect because of the ease with which one can prescribe a medical treatment and

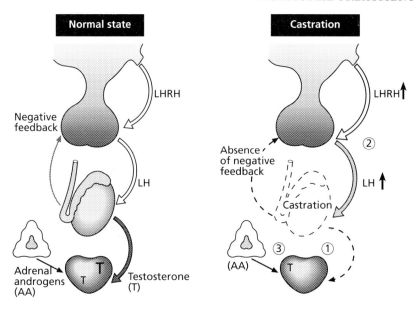

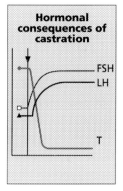

Castration induces *suppression of testicular testosterone* (T) ① (95% of plasma T). This results in a *reactive rise* in LHRH and LH ②.
The 5% of circulating T which persists is derived from the *adrenal glands* ③.
According to some authors, this marked fall in plasma T is not accompanied by a similar fall in intraprostatic dihydrotestosterone (DHT), which remains at about 30% of its initial value (by metabolism of adrenal androgens). This would allow cancer cells very sensitive to DHT to continue to proliferate despite castration. This explains the value, for these authors, of *combined androgenic blockade* which would also block the action of adrenal androgens.

Fig. 3.1 Surgical castration: hormonal consequences. (After Khoury S. *et al.* (1993) *Prostate Cancer Questions (Treatment).* Publication for ICI.)

the automatic follow-up that, in particular, deep injections bring. The review of a patient on a monthly basis for a depot LHRH injection does in fact have many positive advantages in terms of communication and support to the patient, but this has never been quantified. It is our policy to start the majority of patients on a medical form of therapy but following a positive response, to offer substitution of the LHRH agonist by a bilateral orchidectomy. This is usually taken up by the patient after 3 or 4 months when the understanding of their disease has increased and they have begun to notice a gradual atrophy of their testicles due to the medical treatment.

LHRH analogues

LHRH is the hypothalamic hormone responsible for stimulation of hypophyseal gonadotrophic cells. It stimulates the secretion of two gonadotrophins, follicle stimulating hormone (FSH) and luteinizing hormone (LH). LHRH analogues are agonists which have a similar structure to natural LHRH. They reversibly inhibit the production of sex steroids. LHRH is secreted by the hypothalamus and is released directly into the hypothalamo-hypophyseal portal system to act directly on the gonadotrophic cells of the anterior pituitary gland. LHRH binds specifically to membrane receptors situated on the surface of pituitary gonadotrophic cells, this triggers the secretion of LH and FSH. It is important to realize that these LHRH receptors only retain their activity whilst they are intermittently occupied, which is the normal physiological case because LHRH is secreted in a pulsatile manner and has a very short half-life. The use of an LHRH agonist blocks the production of sex steroids by continuously occupying these receptors. The receptors become desensitized, resulting in inhibition of gonadotrophin secretion 10–15 days later. The number of LHRH receptors also decreases during prolonged desensitization.

During this early but important 15-day period, there is a marked rise in LH and FSH because of a more traditional agonist effect. This in turn produces a testosterone flair which may be very dangerous to a patient with potential spinal cord compression from bone metastasis. A sudden rise in testosterone may also put a patient who had until then been only experiencing mild bladder outflow symptoms into acute urinary tension. It is for these reasons that the serum testosterone must be suppressed during this early period, this can be routinely achieved by the use of anti-androgens. These block the testosterone action on target tumour cells, and should be commenced 3 days before the LHRH analogue and continued for the first 4 weeks.

The introduction of LHRH analogues has provided an alternative medical approach to the treatment of advanced prostate cancer, avoiding surgery and its potential complications or the risk of cardiovascular side effects or oestrogen therapy. The LHRH analogues goserelin, leuprolide, tryptorelin and buserelin are registered in many countries for the treatment of prostate cancer. Being peptides, they are susceptible to digestion in the gastrointestinal tract and therefore other routes of administration need to be used to establish sustained plasma concentrations. Injections which have to be given daily and naso-sprays which must be taken several times a day, may be less convenient and less reliable than longer acting depot preparations.

Three of these analogues are available in such depot formations for administration every 28 days and Zoladex has recently been introduced in a 3-monthly depot form. Serum testosterone concentrations are suppressed to the castrate range by 3–4 weeks after the initial administration and remain suppressed provided the drugs are given on a monthly basis. A diagrammatic representation of the action of LHRH analogues is shown in Fig. 3.2.

LHRH analogues produce the expected side effects of testosterone suppression such as hot flushes, loss of libido and impotence. Serious

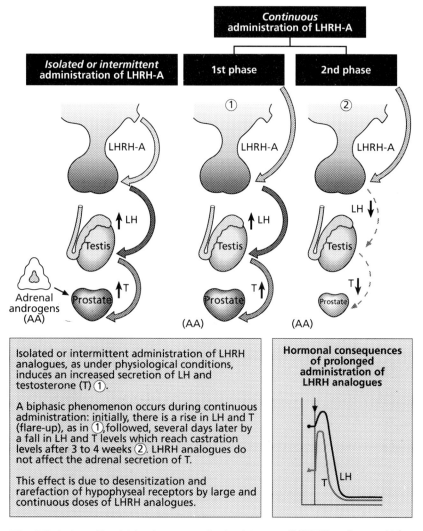

Fig. 3.2 Action of luteinizing hormone-releasing hormone (LHRH) analogues. (After Khoury S. *et al.* (1993) *Prostate Cancer Questions (Treatment)*. Publication for I C I.)

complications only occur when the drugs' initial use has not been protected by a synchronous use of an androgen receptor blocker. Clinicians are becoming increasingly aware that patient choice is an important aspect of treatment and its success. Of two studies in which patients with advanced disease were given a choice between goserelin (Zoladex) or orchidectomy as their initial treatment, 78% of 147 and 86% of 57 patients, respectively, chose Zoladex (Cassileth *et al.* 1989) (Fig. 3.3). The main reasons for this choice were the avoidance of surgery and cosmetic factors. When asked again 3 months later, 93% of the patients and 91% of their wives indicated that they would select the same treatment again.

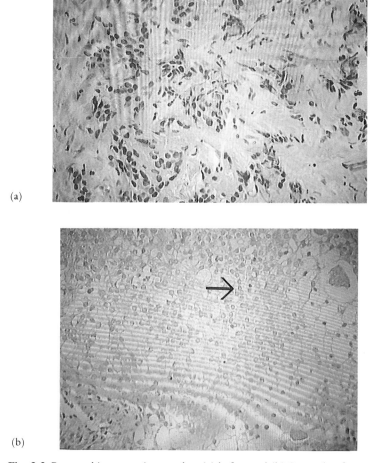

(a)

(b)

Fig. 3.3 Prostate biopsy specimens taken (a) before and (b) 3 months after treatment with an LHRH analogue (Zoladex). Note that whilst most cells are vacuolated and apoptotic, there are some malignant cells seemingly unchanged.

These drugs can conveniently be administered every 4 or 12 weeks with a depot injection into the subcutaneous tissues of the abdominal wall. It is only an observation, but when given by a nurse, a preliminary local anaesthetic is seldom used. The interaction provided by this medical regimen is of great value to a patient with many fears and questions, and is therefore a beneficial side effect.

Hot flushes

Many patients undergoing hormonal treatment for advanced prostate cancer experience hot flushes. Although there are marked differences between the various agents now in clinical use as regards the incidence of this side effect, this disturbance of thermoregulation is still the second most frequent side effect after impotence. Hot flushes are more commonly seen after a bilateral orchidectomy and with the use of LHRH agonist therapy. Hot flushes rarely occur with the use of oestrogens or in monotherapy with the steroidal anti-androgens, such as cyproterone acetate or flutamide. In fact the last two named substances exert a distinct inhibitory effect on hot flushes following treatment with either a bilateral orchidectomy or the use of LHRH agonists. Although these flushes are not dangerous, they can sometimes be extremely bothersome and as a result can potentially reduce the quality of life of patients.

Hot flushes are a symptom of hormone deprivation. There is a close synchrony between the occurrence of a hot flush and an LH pulse. Contrary to long held opinion, the increased gonadotrophin concentration is not responsible for the induction of hot flushes. Hot flushes can also occur in the presence of greatly reduced LH levels, for example in hypophysectomized patients and during LHRH agonist therapy. The primary cause of the disturbance is localized not in the pituitary, but in the hypothalamus. Sex steroids stimulate the release of endogenous opioid peptides in the hypothalamus; these opioids act as inhibitory factors and suppress the intra-hypothalamic release of catecholamines. In turn, catecholamines are the stimulatory neurotransmitter for LHRH secretion. This alternation of inhibitory and stimulatory factors ensures that an increased amount of opioid peptides are released when the sex steroid level is high, as a result of which the catecholamine concentration falls and less LHRH is released. Conversely, small amounts of opioid peptides are released when the sex steroid level is low, leading to an increase in the catecholamine concentration and consequently the increased release of LHRH. In keeping with this regulatory system, the intra-hypothalamic situation in patients suffering from hot flushes is characterized by a decrease of opioids, an increase of catecholamines and an increased LHRH release. Everything now points to the greatly increased concentration of catecholamines as the primary cause of the hot flushes (Casper & Yen 1985). Catecholamines are involved in the physiology regulation of body temperature. Because the mid-brain temperature acts as a thermostat for the regulation of body temperature, the consequence is heat released by the body. Physiologically, a hot flush is an external sign of the activation of heat loss by the body. Both dilatation of the cutaneous vessels and a decrease of the body temperature can be demonstrated as objective signs. This concept should allow the possibility of alleviating hot flushes through the administration of substances such as clonidine which have an inhibitory effect on the central adrenergic activity. This has indeed been demonstrated in a number of studies.

Obviously, the best effect on hot flushes is achieved by replacement therapy with sex steroids. In the case of post-menopausal hot flushes in women, sufficiently high doses of oestrogen lead to complete disappearance of their complaint. Replacement of testosterone in a male with prostate cancer is however contraindicated. It is, however, possible to switch to the administration of progestogens as an alternative. Progestogens are able to release endogenous opioids and in this way exert an inhibitory effect in the regulatory system. The therapeutic effect of replacement with progestogens alone has been demonstrated in a number of clinical studies (Casper & Yen 1985).

The reduction of the testosterone levels secondary to an orchidectomy provokes a counter-regulatory effect with an intra-hypothalamic increase of adrenergic activity from which hot flushes results. The same applies to medical castration with LHRH agonists. The occurrence of hot flushes is not prevented by additional adminstration of pure anti-androgens since these substances have no inhibitory effect on the increased adrenergic activity. A situation similar to that with oestrogen therapy exists in the case of monotherapy with the steroidal anti-androgen cyproterone acetate. This is not only an anti-androgen, but also a potent progestogen and is able to release the hypothalamic inhibitory factors because of this additional activity. The positive effect of these drugs on hot flushes observed in combined therapy after either orchidectomy or administration of LHRH agonists, is attributable to this specific effect on the intra-hypothalamic regulatory mechanism. However, an important practice point is that a lower dose of these anti-androgens is required in combination treatment if their addition is simply to remedy the side effects of hot flushes. The non-steroidal anti-androgens Autamide and Casodex (Zeneca) (see Casodex later) do not have this protective effect as monotherapy but still seem to modify the incidence of hot flushes when used in combination with an LHRH analogue, especially Casodex, and it probably reflects our incomplete understanding of the interaction of these drugs.

Anti-androgens

The mechanism of action of anti-androgens is in competition with androgens for receptor sites within the target organs. An advantage of all well known anti-androgens, in contrast with oestrogen, is the absence of complications regarding the cardiovascular system. Anti-androgens in clinical use for the treatment of advanced prostate cancer can be divided into two types. The first group are the pure anti-androgens (non-steroidal) and the second group are the steroidal anti-androgens; their chemical structures are shown in Fig. 3.4. The level of testosterone in the blood regulates the activity of the hypothalamo-pituitary system by way of a negative feedback on the activity of LHRH-secreting neurones in the hypothalamus (see Fig. 3.5a). Pure anti-androgens (non-steroidal) compete with androgens for receptor sites in the hypothalamus and by doing so stimulate an androgen

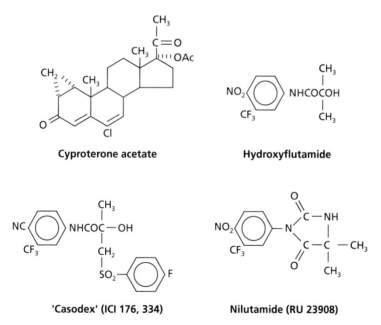

Fig. 3.4 Chemical structures of anti-androgens. Cyproterone acetate is the only steroidal molecule and is not a pure anti-androgen.

deficiency (see Fig. 3.5b). Consequently, more LHRH is released, gona-dotrophin synthesis is stimulated and so is testosterone biosynthesis. Experiments have revealed that this counter-regulatory effect of pure anti-androgens also influences the morphology of the hypothalamus, the pituitary and the testis (Schacher 1981). Within the hypothalamus, there is an increase in the LHRH containing neurones; in the pituitary, the gona-dotrophin producing cells are increased in number and size. The con-sequence of LH secretion is Leydig cell hypoplasia in the testis. As a result of this interference of pure anti-androgens with the hypothalamo-pituitary-gonadal axis, spermatogenesis is not or only partially inhibited and libido, which in males is androgen dependent, is maintained to a certain degree. This latter fact is the great attraction for the use of a pure anti-androgen such as flutamide to be used as monotherapy. However, in contrast to cyproterone acetate, which is a steroidal anti-androgen, it is not possible even with high doses to inhibit prostate weights of intact rats completely (El Etreby et al. 1986). In light of these findings, monotherapy with pure anti-androgens in non-orchidectomized patients or patients already on an LHRH analogue, might entail a certain risk. Steroidal anti-androgens, such as cyproterone acetates (Fig. 3.5c), have a more complex action which in theory is more attractive. These have, in addition to their anti-androgen effects, progesterone-like and anti-gonadotrophic effects. These comple-ment one another in an ideal way by reducing the androgen concentration by inhibition of gonadotrophin secretion, and also inhibiting androgen action within the target organs themselves. This dual mechanism of action explains why complete androgen blockage could in theory be achieved in patients and why it could have been more suitable for monotherapy.

The advantages and disadvantages of these various anti-androgens are summarized in Table 3.1. They can all be used reasonably in combination with either a bilateral orchidectomy or an LHRH analogue as MAB. Many patients are also treated with these anti-androgens as monotherapy but this is only of benefit in those younger patients who wish to retain their potency, and this is only applicable to a pure anti-androgen (non-steroidal) such as Casodex and flutamide.

Cyproterone acetate

When given as daily oral tablets or as intramuscular injections, cyproterone acetate is capable of reducing response with a rate equivalent to that of diethylstilboestrol but with a relatively lower incidence of cardiovascular side effects (De Voogt et al. 1986; Pavone-Macaluso 1986). Several small

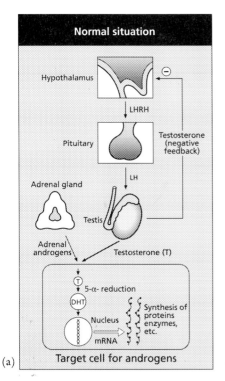

(a)

Fig. 3.5 Regulation of androgen biosynthesis and inhibition of androgen action. (After Schröder F. (ed.) *The Treatment of Prostatic Cancer. Facts and Controversies.* In: EORTC Genitourinary Group, Monograph 8. Wiley-Liss, New York.)

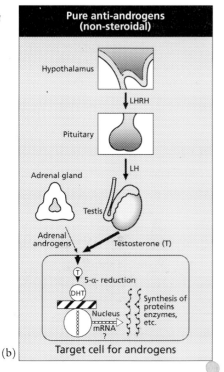

(b)

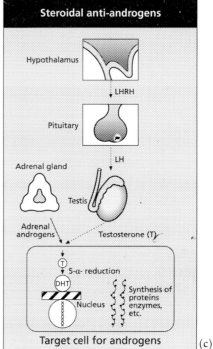

(c)

45

Table 3.1 Inhibition of androgen action.

Regimen	Advantages	Disadvantages
Anti-androgens (general)	Good tolerance as compared with oestrogens Less psychological impact	

Pure anti-androgens	Libido partially maintained
	In combination with castration or LHRH-A:
	    Total androgen blockade
		Suitable for monotherapy?
		Gynecomastia
		In combination with castration or LHRH-A:
		    No inhibition of the initial testosterone peak
		    No effect on hot flushes

Steroidal anti-androgens	Suitable for monotherapy
	Hot flushes only rarely
	In combination with castration or LHRH-A:
	    Total androgen blockade
	In combination with LHRH-A:
	    Inhibition of hot flushes
	    Inhibition of the initial testosterone peak
		Loss of potency

phase two trials have shown an objective response rate of approximately 80% with a mean duration of 17 months and minimal morbidity arising from treatment (Isurugi *et al.* 1980, Tveter 1978). Larger studies have not reproduced such a high response rate but have certainly shown that it is as effective as stilboestrol. The results obtained by the European Organisation of Research on Treatment of Cancer Urological Group were reported by Pavone-Macaluso in 1986. In a randomized phase three trial, the cyproterone acetate (250 mg per day orally) medroxyprogesterone acetate (500 mg by i.m. injection three times per week for 8 weeks followed by a maintenance dose of 200 mg per day orally) and diethylstilboestrol (3 mg per day orally) were compared. In a total of 210 patients with prostate cancer, complete and partial remissions were observed in 33% of the cyproterone acetate treated patients and in 44% of the patients receiving oestrogen; this difference is statistically significant. Local tumour mass reduction of at least 50% was observed and 24 out of 60 of the patients treated with cyproterone acetate. Overall, the incidence of side effects and complications was less in the group receiving cyproterone acetate. There were no significant differences in the cardiovascular death rate of the three treatment groups. However, despite the theoretical advantage in the dual mode action of cyproterone acetate, it has been observed clinically that monotherapy with this drug is unable to suppress gonadotrophin release and androgen production completely; its effect apparently weakens after 6–9 months (Tunn & Thieme 1982). This has led to its combined use with either low dose diethylstilboestrol or with an LHRH analogue in an attempt to produce MAB. It has also been used in patients who relapse after primary hormone therapy on the basis that it may block residual androgens at the target cell level. Smith (1973) treated 35 patients, all of whom had either not responded to oestrogen therapy or who had relapsed afterwards, with 300 mg oral cyproterone acetate daily. Bone pain was reduced in 61% of patients; the size of the prostate was decreased in 43%; and overall subjective and objective improvement was identified in 68% of patients with minimal toxicity and a decrease in the previously oestrogen-induced gynaecomastia, nausea and fluid retention.

Flutamide

The relative affinities of dihydrotestosterone and flutamide clearly show that high concentrations of flutamide are required in order to prevent the access of androgens to the receptor. Thus the weak affinity of flutamide for the dihydrotestosterone (DHT) receptor proteins is a strong argument to always block testicular androgens by medical or surgical castration when using flutamide. Indeed, the observations that about one-third of patients respond to flutamide after failure of medical or surgical castration, whereas no-one responds to castration after failure of flutamide as initial mono-therapy (Sogani et al. 1984; Labrie et al. 1988), suggests that flutamide alone encourages more androgen resistance than castration alone.

Despite this theoretical argument, flutamide has gained a widespread popularity as a form of monotherapy because of its potency and libido preserving effects. Loss of libido and erectile impotence are seen with the use of steroidal anti-androgens, such as cyproterone acetates.

Casodex

Casodex is also a pure and non-steroidal anti-androgen similar in both chemical structure and effect to flutamide. However its distinct advantage is its half-life compatible with once daily oral dosing. In an open phase two study on 267 patients given Casodex, 50 mg/day, an overall objective response (i.e. partial regression) was seen in 55.5% of patients with a further 15.6% having stable disease. However, two of three randomized phase three studies conducted with Casodex 50 mg/day, showed it to be inferior to castration (either medical or surgical) on time to treatment failure and time to progression. A greater fall in serum PSA was observed with Casodex in increasing doses of 100 and 150 mg/day in an open dose ranging study. This suggests that the dose is still not correct for use as monotherapy and current phase three dose escalation studies are underway. All studies do demonstrate its tolerability and minimum side effect profile compared to other non-steroidal anti-androgens, which should make it the natural successor to flutamide as a component of MAB and as monotherapy for younger patients concerned with potency. Potency in an elderly population is seldom respected and lessons can be learned in particular from some of our ethnic minorities of whom continued potency is as important as prolonged survival. This very much changes the clinician's perspective with regard to treatment choices when outcome may be unpredictable.

Intermittent hormone treatment

The reversibility of hormone treatment makes it possible to alternate a patient between elective treatment and no treatment. This approach affords the possibility of recovering sexual function and has been helpful in managing the younger patients with prostate cancer. Professor Oliver recently reported his experience with 17 patients who had requested a short-term stoppage of their treatment. It did not seem unreasonable to allow this and recommend treatment to be restarted when the PSA rose again. The cycles of treatment were generally approximately 6 months in duration and although this was by no means a controlled trial, the impression was that there was no significant alteration in overall survival. There are theoretical advantages in this form of treatment in that the development of hormone resistant cell lines should be diminished if one uses the model of antibiotic resistant bacteria (Akakura *et al.* 1993; Oliver 1994).

Maximum androgen blockade

The concept of maximum androgen blockage (MAB) by eliminating the activity of the adrenal androgens on prostatic cancer cells after castration, was first conceived by Huggins & Scott (1945) 4 years after the publication of their landmark paper on the effects of androgen withdrawal on advanced cancer of the prostate. Their new work showed both a subjective and objective response following bilateral adrenalectomy or hypophysectomy. The high morbidity and mortality decreased the initial enthusiasm, and in clinical research, interest began to focus on the development of drugs able to inhibit the synthesis of adrenal androgens or to block their stimulation at the level of the androgen receptor.

Diethylstilboestrol, orchidectomy and LHRH agonists remarkably suppress 95% of circulating testosterone which represents the output of the testes. However, the weakly androgenic steroids from the adrenal cortex, which are present in the serum in significant concentrations (Coffey 1987), are converted into strong androgens in peripheral tissues such as the prostate (Labrie 1987). Anti-androgens, especially the active metabolite of the non-steroidal agent flutamide, are important as they act as competitive inhibitors for dihydrotestosterone and testosterone receptor proteins, which act on specific DNA sites in the nucleus of the prostate cell. Labrie (1982) was the first to use flutamide and LHRH agonists in an effort to block the effect of the adrenal androgens in the treatment of metastatic prostate cancer.

Bracci was the first to add cyproterone acetate to bilaterial orchidectomy as a first line hormonal treatment in patients with prostate cancer. The promising results stimulated the European Organization for Research and Treatment of Cancer (EORTC) group to launch a phase three trial comparing bilateral orchidectomy bilateral orchidectomy plus cyproterone acetate, and diethylstilboestrol. There was no statistical difference between these three groups (Robinson *et al.* 1988).

The current data on the benefits of MAB is far from conclusion although it does appear to suggest that there is a benefit in terms of prolonging survival times and improving objective response rates compared with monotherapy in patients with minimal disease and good performance status. A meta-analysis is being performed on all the studies employing MAB compared to surgical or medical castration; this will hopefully help to answer the question of its significance. Iversen and colleagues (1990) reported on the Danish prostatic cancer group study. Two hundred and sixty-four patients with locally advanced or metastatic cancer were randomized to receive either orchidectomy or Zoladex plus flutamide and were followed for a median of 39 months (range 29–47 months). Two hundred and sixty-two patients were available for response. In terms of objective response rate, the results were statistically significant in favour over Zoladex plus flutamide, whilst there was no statistically significant difference between the groups in terms of overall survival, timed progression or subjective response rate. Denis and colleagues (1993) reported the results of the EORTC. Three hundred and twenty-seven patients with advanced prostate cancer were randomized to receive orchidectomy, or Zoladex plus flutamide. A significant benefit was seen in combination treatment in terms of disease progression and median survival (mean of 34.4 months versus 27.1 months). Crawford and colleagues (1989) reported on a double blind trial in 603 patients with previously untreated advanced prostate cancer, randomized to receive either leuprolide plus placebo or leuprolide plus flutamide. The parameters used to evaluate the effect of treatment was duration of progression free survival and median length of survival. The difference between the treatments was particularly evident in men with minimal disease and good performance status and there was a statistically significant difference in favour of the MAB group on both parameters.

Side effect profile of maximum androgen blockage

The side effect profile of MAB is greater than for monotherapy except for the bonus of minimizing hot flushes by the use of an anti-androgen with an LHRH analogue. Until recently up to 25% of our patients found MAB intolerable, principally because of gastrointestinal disturbances. Schellhammer (1995) however has recently reported the encouraging results of MAB using Zoladex with Casodex. It is the only study to date, but clearly demonstrates the minimum side effects associated with this combination. Our own small number of patients on this combination also seem to find it as acceptable as monotherapy. Shellhammer compared the efficacy and side effect profile of patients treated with an LHRH analogue combined with flutamide against those treated with the same LHRH analogue and Casodex. There was only a minor advantage in terms of objective progression of disease in favour of the Casodex combination, but there was a dramatic difference with respect to the intolerability caused by diarrhoea. Ten per cent (40/401) experienced diarrhoea on the Casodex combination in contrast to 24% (98/407) on the flutamide combination.

PSA changes following androgen deprivation therapy

When a patient has been started on androgen deprivation therapy, a clinical examination is not necessarily followed by a PSA increase. Because PSA production is androgen dependent, progression may occur without concomitant PSA elevation (Leo et al. 1991). In untreated cases, metastatic disease occurs in less then 2% at a PSA value below 10 mg/ml (Fig. 2.4). In patients relapsing during endocrine therapy, the corresponding value is approximately 30% because the development of hormone resistant disease is not always accompanied by a rise in PSA. In metastatic disease, the bone alkaline phosphates determined by radioimmunoassay, may be more reliable as an indicator of progression, and should be monitored in all patients.

Neoadjuvant hormonal therapy and surgery

Morgan and co-workers (1993) reviewed a series of patients who underwent a radical prostatectomy for clinical stage T3 disease and found a local-recurrence-free 5-year survival rate of 90% compared with 83% for patients treated with post-operative radiation therapy. This is not really a control group, and reflects more the early controlling effects of radiotherapy. The possibilities of metastasing are not mentioned and remain the cause of death in the majority of patients. However, 54% of the patients received adjuvant hormonal therapy confounding the interpretation of the results. Nonetheless, with an overstaging error of 22%, some patients may be cured with radical surgery and adjuvant hormonal manipulation. Moul & Pawson (1991) examined the role of a radical cystoprostatectomy or pelvic exenteration for bulky stage T3 disease. There was a disappointingly high (90%) positive surgical margin rate with a high (50%) serious complication rate including a 40% re-operation rate. However, because of the bulk extent of the cancer in these selected patients, these results represent treatment for those patients at the adverse end of the spectrum of stage T3 disease. Cystoprostatectomy for non-bulky clinical stage T3 disease as monotherapy has not been adequately studied, but one must be circumspect given the obvious microscopic findings of inadequate hormone treatment of T3 prostate cancers by a neoadjuvant 3 month course of an LHRH analogue (Fig. 3.3).

Early or delayed hormonal treatment?

The timing of hormonal therapy has been an issue almost more controversial than the type of hormonal therapy itself. Clinicians have always been more ready to start a treatment early in a relatively young patient and delay that same treatment in a much older individual. Several studies now point to the improved effects in terms of increased survival and delay of progression with immediate hormonal therapy. The study that started this controversy did not have this issue as its objective. An unexpected result of the first Veterans Administration Co-operative Urological Research Group (VACURG) study was that patients randomized to the placebo arm were allowed to remain in the study although they required hormone treatment because of disease progression with pain. After 9 years, all patients on the placebo arm had received some form of hormonal treatment and this inadvertent decision has shown that their survival rate was not different from patients randomized to treatment arms from the beginning of the study (Blackard & Byar 1972). One possible conclusion from this was that delaying hormonal treatment did not shorten survival and, if one considers palliative treatment, then this could begin when symptoms arrive which would be not only more economical, but also reduce the morbidity or length of duration of possible side effects from the treatment.

There is, by contrast, an hypothesis that immediate treatment should at least be indicated for those with a larger volume of metastasis. It has been found that the larger volume of metastasis is linked to a shorter survival and is usually more difficult to treat. In an experimental study, Isaacs (1984) demonstrated, by using the Downing tumour module, that castration at the time of tumour innoculation led to a longer survival as opposed to delayed castration. The first VACURG study demonstrated that placebo treated patients with an 8-year follow-up had an almost 50% higher probability of stage progression compared to patients with hormonal therapy. Finally, patients submitted for observation only for late prostatic carcinoma could develop undesirable complications of their cancer, such as pathological bone fractures, earlier than would occur if stage progression could be delayed by treatment although this has never been proved. In essence, although delaying treatment is probably only justified in asymptomatic, elderly (over 70 years old) patients with advanced prostate cancer, at the time of diagnosis there are good arguments for immediate hormone manipulation. On reviewing all our patients where the decision was not clear cut and the patient was given as much information as possible, the request by 88% of patients was to start treatment immediately. This is a much more reasonable approach now that new drug modalities have been developed that are associated with a low grade side effect profile.

The first major report on the use of hormonal treatment for prostate cancer was by Nesbit (1950). One thousand eight hundred and eighteen cases were compared with a historical series of cases collected between 1925 and 1940; these latter cases were nominally called the controls. For those patients who had presented with metastases, the 5-year survival was 44% compared to 10% for the control group. There was no significant difference between the method of hormonal manipulation. For those patients pre-senting with metastases, the 5-year survival was 20% compared with 6% for controls. Therefore, there appeared to be a survival advantage for the use of early hormonal treatment, with a clear advantage for non-metastatic or low volume metastatic disease.

This study very much dictated the strategy for the majority of urologists and until two decades later when three consecutive studies from the VACURG reported their results using much more controlled data. The results of the VACURG studies have been reviewed many times, but Chisholm (1990) has succinctly stated that there are three points from this work that are relevant in any discussion of current attitudes to the early treatment of prostate cancer. The first was the demonstration of the hazards of high dose oestrogen, which led to attempts to define the optimum lower dose. A second observation from a following study (Byar 1972) was that those treated with either placebo or low dose (0.2 mg per day) stilboestrol had a greater progression to stage IV disease compared with those receiving either 1 mg or 5 mg stilboestrol daily. The third and much more quoted observation was that there was no disadvantage in terms of survival by delaying treatment for those with asymptomatic disease. This conclusion was further supported by a report from Lepor and co-workers (1982) who compared the survival of 65 patients with advanced prostate cancer treated between 1937 and 1940, i.e. before the introduction of hormone therapy, to the survival of 47 similar patients treated with hormonal manipulation between 1942 and 1943. After accounting for the changing patterns of survival from one decade to the next, these authors could find no statistically significant survival benefit from early hormone treatment.

One can understand from these later reports why the tide of opinion was in support of delayed treatment. However, both clinicians and patients have always been uncomfortable with this concept and careful reanalysis of previous studies suggest that whilst there is no benefit overall, there would be a benefit of early hormonal treatment for those patients with low volume disease. The main reasons for recommending early hormone treatment for all forms of locally advanced prostate cancer (patients with locally advanced disease, with and without metastases, that may or may not be symptomatic), are as discussed below.

• It is a general oncological principle that it is better to treat any tumour when it is small rather than large and there is no reason why prostate cancer should be an exception. This is even supported by the VACURG study (Byar 1977) and the American College of Surgeons' survival data (Mettlin et al. 1982).

• Local progression of a prostate cancer will quite often require a second channel transurethral resection in someone whose initial hormone treatment has been deferred. This is not seen in patients who are started on early treatment.

- There is also a need for a better definition of asymptomatic disease. The absence of bone pain is very subjective, more subtle adverse effects such as anaemia, weight loss, blood dyscrasia, oedema, ureteric obstruction and general malaise may be disturbing to the patient's lifestyle. The fact that these problems occur without the patient being aware of them is well illustrated by the positive, subjective improvement, commonly noted by patients after they start hormone treatment. It would not be unreasonable to give the patients a chance of avoiding some of these adverse systemic effects by the early treatment of their cancer. It is unfortunate that quality of life issues have only attracted scientific attention more recently. It has always been quite clear to clinicians that the majority of patients prefer to feel that something is being done about their cancer and find it hard to subject themselves to the observation, no matter how close and caring it is. Robinson (1988) has commented that elderly patients suffering from prostate cancer were more concerned about their ability to lead a normal life and to support their families than about their disease, status and probable length of survival. The greatest factor that affects quality of life is anxiety and this is substantially decreased when treatment is started.

- Local prostate complications are ultimately fewer after treatment (28%).

- Deferred treatment is often associated with local progression which may cause ureteral and/or bladder outlet obstruction. In a study by Avs (1995), 61% of 514 patients with prostate cancer needed one or more palliative surgical procedures before death, and an average of 5 weeks was spent in hospital due to prostate cancer.

Although our policy in this department is to recommend the treatment of asymptomatic advanced cancer in patients with an otherwise expected survival of 10 years by hormonal manipulation, and where tolerated, with MAB, there is still the need for a definitive controlled study; this has been addressed by the Medical Research Council (MRC). This study which started in 1985 and closed in 1993 (Kirk 1985, 1987), included any patient with histologically proven, advanced localized or metastatic disease, for whom there was genuine doubt as to whether hormone treatment was immediately required, was eligible for randomization either to immediate hormone treatment or to delayed treatment until a specific indication arose. The data from this trial is still very much immature and prevents any final conclusion being drawn. However, some interesting points are already apparent (Kirk 1993). For example, local prostatic tumour progression is as common a reason for treatment of those initially randomized to deferred treatment as is metastatic disease. Although those with metastasis require treatment sooner, 40% of patients with M1 disease are untreated at 1 year.

Unlike the VACURG studies, in the MRC study the majority of deaths are from prostate cancer and not from other causes; this feature has a consensus view given the overall increased age at which our patients are living.

Despite improvements in the methods of administering hormone treatment, there are still significant side effects which must be borne in mind when starting hormonal treatment early. The cost of such hormone treatment now means that the majority of patients are receiving medical treatment rather than orchidectomy, and the number continues to escalate. If immediate treatment continues to show a benefit in terms of survival or prevention of complications, there would be a clear wave of concern in those more concerned with health economics. One compromise, which must not be lightly dismissed, might have to be a trend back towards an orchidectomy under local anaesthesia complemented by the use of an anti-androgen such as Casodex, which would halve the relevant budget. Delay in progression of disease and an increase in survival time are not unreasonable objectives while we await the ultimate cure. Early treatment of low volume disease by MAB seems to have provided this compromise but the evidence is not uniform. Given the diagnosis of malignant disease, the majority of patients wish to achieve treatment. This would be acceptable if it was not for the fact that some advanced prostate cancers are so slow growing that treatment is not required – at least for as long as expected survival is not altered by advances in health and health care in general – and that such hormonal treatment may have unpleasant side effects. The side effects of MAB have been reduced with the introduction of new anti-androgens. But the cornerstone of management, in the absence of a definitive cure, is data on quality of life issues. Controlled comparative trials using quality outcome measures are in progress and we eagerly await the results.

Finasteride

Finasteride has been the first 5-alpha reductase inhibitor to be evaluated in the human. Clinical studies in normal volunteers and patients with benign prostatic hyperplasia (BPH) have established that treatment with finasteride results in a significant decrease in both serum and intra-prostatic dihydrotestosterone (DHT). Serum testosterone levels are slightly elevated whereas intra-prostatic levels are markedly increased. However, serum and intra-prostatic levels of PSA are decreased, suggesting that the elevated testosterone levels have little or no biological function in the prostate once 5-alpha reductase is inhibited. The as yet unproved theory is that malignant prostate tissue may also retain this selectivity. This in turn, not only raises the possibility of finasteride as a therapy for prostate cancer, but also suggests that its prolonged use in patients with BPH may possibly be protective against the development of prostate cancer. This is highly speculative but makes it essential for us to follow our patients on finasteride closely, carrying out a transrectal ultrasound (TRUS) and perhaps even a random biopsy, if there is any fluctuation in the patients' free/total PSA ratio.

Hormone resistant disease

Patients who fail to respond to primary ablation of testicular androgens must do so either because the cancer includes an androgen independent clone of cells, or alternatively a clone which is super-sensitive to androgen has been selected and has become the dominant cancer line. If minimally androgen dependent clones do prevail, stimulation by adrenal androgens could support continued cellular growth. This is a form of what I have called 'cellular sociology' and may also involve active communication between cells, passing on 'resistance' information. If this is the case then suboptimal treatment such as inadequate testosterone suppression or radiotherapy may be actively encouraging the development of resistant cancer.

A rise in PSA is an otherwise asymptomatic patient should prompt a bone scan, abdomen ultrasound and chest X-ray. Such a rise in PSA, which is the earliest marker of a hormone resistant cancer, should not in itself be a reason for changing the patient's treatment. Even if a significant metastasis is identified on the evaluation, there is still no indication for local treatment. Even local radiotherapy for a bone metastasis may contribute to a relative degree of marrow suppression with the only advantage being bio-chemical in that the PSA may be lowered. Survival cannot be influenced by such interference and so in these cases, the rising PSA remains an enigma that both clinicians and now patients can find uncomfortable. Patients have a far greater insight into their health and in particular into the PSA test to which they attach an almost magical importance since many of them blame the test or their diagnosis in the first place. Coming to terms with a rising PSA and a clinician that does not seem to want to do anything new can cause anxiety. A holistic and necessary approach starts with a frank discussion concerning the outcome of their disease at the time of diagnosis. A counsellor or palliative care nurse has an important role in this setting. The busy outpatient department is not an ideal setting to discuss the rest of the patient's life, and we have found that specialized clinics help this communication dilemma. Patient's awareness and education has also been transformed by the use of a record chart that the patient keeps and brings with him to his clinic. This is also available for any visiting nurse or when the patient may be on vacation. This will be discussed fully in Chapter 5.

Chemotherapy

Whilst it is recognized that there is a high initial response rate to hormonal treatment, most patients will eventually have progressive disease with a median survival from the discovery of distant metastases to death remaining in the range of 1–3 years (Whitmore *et al.* 1972). In spite of the need for more effective systemic therapies, the introduction of cytotoxic chemotherapy in the treatment of prostate cancer has been a slow and difficult process. The use has very much been limited to patients with hormone resistant disease who may have also received radiotherapy. These patients are of an advanced age, generally have a low performance status and may have subclinical marrow suppression which altogether make them a very difficult group on which to imagine chemotherapy might have a reasonable effect.

Before 1973, very few non-hormonal chemotherapeutic agents had been tested in prostate cancer (Yagoda *et al.* 1972). Several single agents, when administered to patients after response failure to hormone treatment, appear to have only a modest activity in this disease.

Cisplatin is one of the most extensively evaluated agents. Merrin & Beckley (1979) employed a weekly schedule at a dose of 1 mg/kg for 6 consecutive weeks and they reported an encouraging overall response rate of 31% with stabilization of the disease in an additional 26% of hormone resistant patients. However, in five subsequent studies performed at the Memorial Hospital (Yagoda & Vurgrin 1979), a much more modest rate of responses was demonstrated with a cumulative response of only 5%. Even this effect must be offset by the significant potential for severe toxicity in this patient population.

Cyclophosphamide and doxorubicin have also proved to be unremarkable when used as single agents unless one is attracted by the relatively unscientific parameter of disease stabilization. Other conventional agents that appear to have some activity on hormone resistant prostate cancer include 5-fluorouracil (Chlebowski *et al.* 1977), hydroxyurea (Mundy 1982), and methotrexate (Loening *et al.* 1983). Recent trials with two additional conventional drugs have demonstrated moderately encouraging results. The vinblastine, at a dose of 1.5 mg/m^2/day for 5 days produced 21% partial response rate with limited toxicity. An EORTC study

Table 3.2 Randomized single agent studies in hormone resistant prostatic cancer. (From Hesketh P.J. In: Fitzpatrick J., Krane R. (eds) *The Prostate*. Churchill Livingstone, Edinburgh.)

Reference	Treatment*	Patients		Response†		Median Survival‡
		Total	Evaluable	CR+PR	SD	
Scott (1976)	CTX	—	41	4	20	47
	5-FU	—	33	4	14	44
	Standard	—	36	0	7	38
Schmidt (1979)	CTX	39	35	0	9	27
	DTIC	68	55	2	13	40
	Procarbazine	58	39	0	5	31
Loening (1981)	CTX	47	43	3	12	41
	MeCCNU	38	27	1	7	22
	Hydroxyurea	40	28	2	2	19
deWys (1983)	Doxorubicin	112	61	15	—	29
	5-FU	54	42	3	—	24
Tejada (1977)	5-FU	9	8	2	1	NS
	CCNU	10	10	4	2	NS
Pavone-Macaluso (1980)	Doxorubicin	22	11	0	3	NS
	Procarbazine	24	14	1	0	NS

* CTX, cyclophosphamide; 5-FU, 5-fluorouracil; DTIC, dacarbazine; MeCCNU, methylcyclohexylnitrosourea.
† CR, complete; PR, partial; SD, stable disease.
‡ Expressed in weeks; NS, not stated.

employing a mitomycin-c at a dose of $15\,mg/m^2$ intravenously every 6 weeks demonstrated a partial response of 29% in 31 patients, again with limited toxicity. Several new cytotoxic agents have been screened for activity in prostate cancer but negligible activity has been noted. Table 3.2 summarizes the randomized single agent studies in hormone resistant prostate cancer.

An appreciable number of clinical trials have been performed in an attempt to improve upon the modest results of single agent chemotherapy in hormone resistant prostate cancer by using combinations of the most active drugs. However, there has been no conclusive evidence to date that combinations of these drugs are superior to single drugs in this disease. Much of the enthusiasm surrounding the initial reports of promising combination drug schemes in the non-randomized trials, is tempered by review of the randomized studies comparing single drug and multiple agent chemotherapy. In the eight randomized studies shown in Table 3.3, no difference in survival has been observed between single drug and combination therapy. In addition, with the exception of the study by Stephens and colleagues (1984), no statistical advantage for combination chemotherapy with respect to the response rate has been demonstrated.

Combined chemotherapy and hormone treatment

A concept of combining cytotoxic drugs with hormonal manipulation in prostate cancer is conceptionally very attractive because of the different mechanisms of action of these modalities and their non-overlapping toxicities. Histological evaluation of prostate cancer following hormonal treatment shows that the majority of cells have not reached apoptosis but are severely swollen (Civantos 1995). The desire to push these cells into apoptosis with the use of proven cytotoxic drugs is very attractive. Isaacs (1984), employing the transplantable rat prostate tumour model, has produced experimental evidence of the potential superiority of early aggressive multi-agent intervention in prostate cancer. His group have found firstly, that androgen ablation therapy or cyclophosphamide therapy employed singularly is most effective when started early, but neither is curative, and secondly, that the combination of cyclophosphamide and androgen ablation is more effective than either alone, and the earlier the administration the greater the survival. Attempts to clinically validate this study have had mixed results. Oestramustine, a synthetic drug combining oestradiol and the alkylating agent nitrogen mustard, has been shown to have appreciable activity when used in previously untreated prostate cancer

Table 3.3 Randomized studies comparing single agent versus combination chemotherapy in hormone resistant prostate cancer. (From Hesketh P.J. In: Fitzpatrick J., Krane R. (eds) *The Prostate*. Churchill Livingstone, Edinburgh.)

References	Drug*	Patients Total	Evaluable	Response† CR	PR	SD	I	Response criteria‡	Median survival
Herr (1982)	CCNU	20	20	0	0	6		NPCP	24 weeks
	vs CTX+MTX+5-FU	20	20	0	3	4			26 weeks
Chlebowski (1978)	CTX	15	15	0	0	8		NPCP	7.2 months
	vs CTX+DOX+5-FU	12	12	0	0	6			8.9 months
Muss (1981)	CTX	21	17	0	0	9		NPCP	8 months
	vs CTX+MTX+5-FU	19	15	0	1	7			5.2 months
Kasimis (1985)	CTX	16	16	0	0	8		NPCP	NS
	vs 5-FU+DOX+MITO-C	15	14	0	1	5			
Torti (1985)	DOX	20	15	0	0	8		NPCP	48 weeks
	vs DOX+DDP	17	17	0	1	9		ASS	43 weeks
Eagen (1976)	DOX	19	19	0	0	0	5		NS
	vs CTX+5-FU	18	18	0	0	0	2		NS
Smalley (1981)	5-FU	49	29	0	0	14		SECG	34.4 weeks
	vs CTX+DOX+5-FU	52	29	0	0	20			25.2 weeks
Stephens (1984)	Hydroxyurea	158	69	0	1/24	—		S	28 weeks
	vs CTX+DOX		68	1/19	5/19	—			27 weeks

* CCNU, cyclohexylnitrosourea; CTX, cyclophosphamide; MTX, methotrexate; 5-FU, fluorouracil; DOX, doxorubicin; MITO-C, mitomycin-C; DDP, cisplatin.
† CR, complete; PR, partial; SD, stable disease; I, improvement.
‡ NPCP, National Prostatic Cancer Project; ASS, Ancillary Scoring System; SECG, Southeastern Cancer Group; S, Usual Criteria for Solid Tumours; NS, not stated.

patients with objective response rates of up to 90% (Slack 1979). Several non-randomized phase two studies that combined additional cytotoxic agents and hormonal treatment as the initial treatment for metastatic prostate cancer have been reported. Previous studies, employing the combination of bilateral orchidectomy with stilboestrol and cisplatin, noted partial regression in 66% of patients, with 17% of patients achieving stable disease. One of the most interesting series using a combined chemo/hormonal approach was reported by Servadio and colleagues (1983) where patients initially underwent bilateral orchidectomy followed by stilboestrol at a dose of 3 mg/day and weekly intravenous cylophosphamide (10 mg/kg) and 5-fluorouracil (10 mg/kg) for 2 years. In the third year, the dose of the latter two drugs was reduced by 50% and they were given every 3 weeks. For patients still under treatment by the fifth year, both drugs were administered every 4 weeks. Bone scans stabilized or improved in 79% of patients and elevated acid phosphatase levels were reduced to normal levels in 80% of cases. Pain relief was achieved in 75% of patients. The most impressive result was a 6-year survival rate of 50% of patients.

Unfortunately, phase three trials have not confirmed these early exciting results. Murphy and co-workers (1983, 1986) showed no significant difference with respect to response rate or survival between orchidectomy alone, oestramustine alone or a combination of cyclophosphamide plus 5-

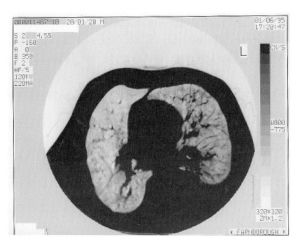

Fig. 3.6 CT scan showing lymphangitis carcinomatosis in a patient with hormone resistant prostate cancer. He presented with breathing difficulties and his symptoms could only be palliated with high dose prednisolone. Chemotherapy produced a short term symptomatic improvement, but subsequently made him susceptible to a fatal opportunistic pneumonia.

fluorouracil plus stilboestrol. The attractive concept of combined treatment looks to have a bleak future. Its only remaining potential that was evident in Isaac's (1984) rat model was one of early intervention with this treatment. Such a loophole seems unlikely given that clinical responses by other solid tumours to systemic treatment show success even in relapsed or late disease.

One alternative and very opposite potential strategy may be to strangely increase the testosterone levels prior to chemotherapy. Prostatic cancer is characteristically slow growing and thus insensitive to cytotoxic agents, which are most active against rapidly proliferating cells. If prostatic cancer growth could be transiently stimulated, perhaps by hormonal meals, concurrently administered cytotoxic agents might potentially be more active. In our prospective controlled clinical trial (Manni *et al.* 1985), androgen 'priming' was used with cytotoxic therapy in hormone resistant cancer. The results were encouraging in the short term, but there was ultimately no difference in response duration or survival. In addition, several patients in the testosterone 'priming' group developed severe symptoms such as pain or even spinal cord compression and were withdrawn from the study.

When a patient has failed hormone treatment, radiotherapy in the form of hemibody irradiation, and if focal treatment or systemic intravenous treatment has been used to the point of potential marrow toxicity, there remains little in favour of exposing a patient to the side effects of chemotherapy (Fig. 3.6). It is a natural desire by both patients and their families to request that all possible is done. But for the sake of the patient's dignity (and their income and marital status), the role of chemotherapy should be played down. Correct information and treatment must be offered but with the strong recommendation that the 'cure', if any, is much worse than the disease.

Practice points

• Neoadjuvant hormonal treatment of T0–T2 disease possibly of value. T3 disease is not down-staged.

• Early use of maximum androgen blockage for low volume metastatic disease in those aged under 70 years (this includes T3, N0 and M0 disease) will probably increase survival and delay progression of either local or metastatic disease. There remains the disadvantage of significant medical side effects in at least 20% of these patients. The patient should be aware of these choices.

• Delayed hormonal treatment is appropriate for asymptomatic advanced disease in those over 70 years. Monotherapy with a 3 month depot LHRH analogue (covered by short term anti-androgen cover) is suitable for symptomatic advanced disease. The addition of an anti-androgen often produces a positive secondary effect. These drugs are expensive and a bilateral orchidectomy must be considered a reasonable alternative as a first line hormonal treatment in some health care economies.

• A rise in serum PSA whilst on hormone treatment indicates developing resistance but because this may precede symptomatic disease by up to 2 years there is not an indication to alter treatment. There is however an indication to reinvestigate the patient with a bone scan and spinal MRI.

• Combined chemotherapy and hormonal treatment has no practical value. Chemotherapy for hormone resistant disease is often greeted with enthusiasm by a patient and his relatives but controlled trials do not support its value and whilst it should be offered, this must be undertaken with a realistic pessimism.

Chapter 4
Treatment of Local Disease

Prostatism

Prostatism is an umbrella term that encompasses the symptoms of bladder outflow obstruction (hesitancy, poor stream, terminal dribbling) and bladder irritability (frequency, urgency, nocturia). This cluster of symptoms occurs in patients with advanced prostate cancer either because of outflow obstruction with secondary irritative symptoms, or because of primary irritation caused by infiltration of the bladder trigone by the cancer. Sometimes, of course, there is a combination of both pathophysiological processes taking place, but generally the specific symptomatology of the patient will point to one of these two underlying mechanisms. In particular, symptoms of bladder irritability caused by trigone infiltration will respond very well to hormone manipulation with or without radiotherapy, but will respond poorly to any form of palliative surgery. This is a not dissimilar situation to the lessons that we have learnt in the management of benign prostatic hyperplasia (BPH) and the need to choose the right patients for surgery.

The incidence of pure bladder outflow obstruction in patients with advanced prostate cancer has begun to decrease at the time of presentation because, in general, the disease has been discovered much earlier than in the past. Sixty per cent of patients were said to have significant obstructive symptoms at the time of presentation in an investigative study. However the majority of patients with advanced prostate cancer who may not present with significant symptoms in contemporary times will eventually develop them as their disease slowly progresses. Assessment of outflow obstruction should involve a close attention to how bothersome are the symptoms to the patient, and at least one flow rate evaluation should be performed. The value of a post-micturition residual assessment is of the same relative value as when diagnosing outflow obstruction due to BPH. I do not think that there is a place for full urodynamic studies in these patients when symptoms of bladder irritability predominate, because the confirmation of suspected trigonal infiltration will come with the response to hormonal manipulation that the patient should be put on.

There is no absolute indication for a transurethral resection other than the presence of urinary retention. A transurethural resection of the prostate (TURP) should not be performed to gain more tissue for histology; it is not that unusual for the histological assessment of tissue from the channel resection in a patient with known prostate cancer to be negative because the cancer is confined to the untouched periphery of the gland. If further histological assessment is required, then a transrectal biopsy should be performed under ultrasound control. In those individual cases where hormonal manipulation is delayed, a TURP may be indicated for bothersome outflow symptoms. This usually takes the form of a channel TURP: a limited channel is resected because this produces the same functional results as a wider resection, but recognizes the fact that regrowth of peripheral; tissue is not an issue over the same time span as when this operation is done for BPH. However, this is not strictly true, and if there is one operation that many urologists prefer not to do it is a second revision channel TURP, because of the altered anatomical landmarks due to a combination of prostatic regrowth and malignant infiltration. Hence there is a responsibility to carry out an adequate resection in the first instance, particularly if the patient has a good prognosis from their prostate cancer.

Many patients with locally advanced cancer have traditionally received radiotherapy which will stabilize and control future symptoms. This is not the practice in our department, but many patients do come to us having received this treatment. Some of these patients will continue to experience symptoms of outflow obstruction or indeed may develop them *de novo* as a result of the radiotherapy. This latter group of patients include strictures at the bladder neck and in the urethra as a result of irradiation. These problems occur in approximately 20% of patients who undergo the radiation, with a slightly increased risk if there have been significant outflow symptoms prior to radiotherapy. A significant number of patients with outflow obstruction are helped by local radiotherapy but the problem is that post-radiotherapy surgery is not always straightforward. The resection of prostatic tissue that has received radiotherapy is often associated with a more significant blood loss peri-operatively and a high incidence of post-operative bladder neck stenosis (20%). It is for these reasons that we prefer not to use radiotherapy for patients with symptoms of prostatism unless the majority of the patients' symptoms are those of bladder irritability, and hormonal manipulation for one reason or another is not acceptable.

Several authors have expressed concern over the possible role of TURP in the dissemination of prostate cancer (Bandhauer 1975; Hanks *et al.* 1983). However, further studies have quite clearly shown that the majority of patients in previous trials who underwent a TURP, and subsequently had a shorter time to progression of their disease, were patients of a much poorer prognosis with a higher grade and stage of disease upon presentation. This followed a general trend where patients with more advanced disease underwent a transurethral resection, and those with a more limited disease underwent hormonal manipulation. This argument is of less relevance today in the light of molecular staging which shows that 95% of patients with clinical locally advanced disease have potential micro-metastases in their blood stream. The theoretical question as to whether any surgical or therapeutic procedure reduces the general immune status of the patient and so allows a micro-metastasis to further develop must remain unanswered for the moment, but it is unlikely to alter the management of our patients.

Cryosurgery is the *in situ* destruction of a tumour by the application of low temperatures. It was first developed in the late 1970s to treat localized prostate cancer (Addonizio 1982), but it was associated with a great number of complications and a low level of ultimate cure that may have been due to understaging but could quite likely be also due to inadequate treatment (Bonney 1978). New devices have been developed which more closely monitor the temperatures produced and so can avoid the previously reported side effects.

Successful animal studies of the new technology has prompted evaluation of a percutaneous transperineal prostate cryosurgery procedure guided by transrectal ultrasound (TRUS). A number of facts became apparent through this early experience. First, placing one or two probes a number of times into the prostate was not adequate to destroy all the abnormal tissue reliably, and secondly, a new system with at least cryoprobes that could be used simultaneously would be needed. However the procedure is well tolerated and associated with minimal morbidity. The previously reported high incidence of urethrorectal fistulae and urethrocutaneous fistulae has not been apparent. This work is still very much in its developmental phase but it does seem reasonable that it will have a role in the control of locally advanced disease when, for various reasons, a patient cannot or does not want to undergo a channel TURP. I do not think that it has a role in the treatment of localized disease because we will only see a repeat of the earlier poor results in line with our frustration in dealing with understaged localized disease by all other forms of treatment.

Urinary retention

Approximately 13% of patients who present in urinary retention have a diagnosis of locally advanced prostate cancer (Moul *et al.* 1989). This figure is similar to facts from our own department from a similar time, but in the last 5 years this figure has fallen to 5%. Initial treatment of these patients can involve either a channel TURP or hormonal manipulation, or both. A channel TURP has the advantage of early restoration of normal micturition but is not without morbidity, particularly in a slightly increased age group when compared to those presenting with urinary retention caused by BPH. Previous studies (Fleishmann *et al.* 1985) have suggested that hormonal manipulation alone is a preferable treatment for patients with locally advanced prostate cancer and urinary retention. Clinically many of these patients will have a varying volume of cancer and it is sometimes impossible to determine whether the cancer alone has been the cause of the urinary retention. Concomitant BPH is always present.

In one study reported by Thomas and colleagues (1992), a controlled trial was performed between two groups of patients. One group underwent a channel TURP and bilateral orchidectomy and the second group underwent a bilateral orchidectomy alone. The only morbidity occurred in the channel TURP group where two patients required blood transfusion and one patient suffered a severe urinary tract infection. Four patients out of ten failed to void spontaneously immediately following a channel TURP and required recatheterization for a number of months. A subsequent trial without catheter in these patients was successful. This is in contrast to the second group of patients where hormonal treatment alone was given. In this group, the catheter was routinely left *in situ* for 1 month. Two out of 12 patients failed to void in this group and these underwent a successful channel TURP. Despite the small size of this study it is quite clear that this group of patients have an unpredictable outcome following immediate surgery, and hormonal manipulation is associated with much less morbidity both in the short and long term. Ultimately a channel TURP may be needed in patients who have begun hormonal manipulation, but these will be in the minority and will hopefully be in a more elective and controlled setting.

Haematuria and haemorrhage

Many papers that support the concept of radical surgery for the attempted cure of localized prostate cancer cite the small incidence in subsequent local symptoms to be further justification of this treatment. I am certainly an advocate of such surgery when the cancer is proved to be truly localized and the patient has an expected survival of over 10 years. I am not impressed by the concept of controlling local symptoms, because such symptoms are indeed rare in the typical practice of a urologist in the UK where radical surgery has rarely been employed. Local symptoms have been adequately controlled with either radiotherapy and/or hormonal manipulation, and the number of patients presenting with either intractable perineal pain or haemorrhage are very few and amount to no more than 0.5% of our prostate cancer patients in any one year. However, when a local problem such as haemorrhage does occur it can be very difficult to treat. A review of our last three cases has shown that this has occurred in hormone resistant disease, but not necessarily in the terminal phase of their disease. In each of these cases there was not a demonstrable bleeding or clotting disorder, but the known association of metastatic prostate cancer with the production of fibrinolytic compounds has been established (Adamson *et al.* 1994), making medical management unlikely. As with all associated ailments for a cancer patient, it demands not just prompt attention, but also a solution that returns the patient to 'normality' quickly.

Endoscopic coagulation has been uniformly unsuccessful in the longer term and the patient spends a protracted period in hospital forlornly waiting for the haemorrhage to settle. It is rare for a specific bleeding site to be identified on an arteriogram and this may be due to a lack of contrast extravasation in the presence of active bleeding caused by chronic capillary bleeding from a broad surface of hypervascular granulation tissue formed in response to radiation or from hypervascular neoplastic tissue (Higgins 1977). Traditionally bilateral embolization, even of the internal iliac arteries, has been required due to the extensive collateral network from the external iliac, common femoral and inferior mesenteric arteries (Mitchell 1976). However, superselective arterial catheterization of the combined prostatic and inferior vesical branches, carried out by a Seldinger technique, is to be preferred. The origin of the prostatovesical artery is variable, more commonly arising from the gluteopudendal trunk, and less commonly arising from the umbilical, internal pudendal or obturator arteries (Clegg 1955). Embolization with gel-foam has proved to be universally successful in our hands and is to be recommended as a first choice treatment when hormonal treatment and radiotherapy have been previously used. This distal embolization is not associated with buttock pain and the patient can be mobilized on the following day.

Practice points

• Prostatism will respond to hormonal treatment. Over two thirds of patients in urinary retention secondary to prostate cancer can avoid a transurethral resection of the prostate (TURP) if hormonal treatment alone is used.

• Cryosurgery is a complicated and a slightly more hazardous alternative to a TURP.

• Haematuria in a patient with hormone resistant disease can sometimes be successfully treated by transurethal coagulation. Local radiotherapy or super selective embolization should be used in failed cases.

• A TURP in a patient within 12 months of radical radiotherapy is associated with greater morbidity and should be avoided if possible by using hormonal treatment.

Chapter 5
Treatment of Metastatic Disease

Ureteric obstruction

The incidence of unilateral upper tract obstruction in advanced prostate cancer is not uncommon but when partial is usually asymptomatic because of its chronic insidious onset. It can be diagnosed on a bone scan by the appearance of delayed secretion of isotope from the affected kidney. A review of 250 bone scans at King's College Hospital over the last 5 years has demonstrated a bilateral hydronephrosis in 20 (8%) patients and a unilateral hydronephrosis in 56 (24%) patients. Fifty per cent and 95% respectively of these were in asymptomatic patients although close scrutiny of the serum creatinine in those patients with bilateral hydronephrosis demonstrated mild renal failure in all cases. A significant post-micturition residual can also be identified on such a bone scan (Fig. 5.1) and this occurred in 30% of those without upper tract dilatation and 66% in association with patients with upper tract obstruction. This latter combination is caused by prostatic cancer extension towards the trigone and this can often feel so flat and smooth on rectal examination that the diagnosis is missed by many non-urological specialists. Ureteric obstruction can also be caused by paranodal lymphatic disease and this is the main cause of a unilateral obstruction without associated bladder outflow obstruction (Fig. 5.2).

The therapeutic options available for management of ureteric obstruction associated with prostate cancer include the following alternatives:
1 no treatment;
2 hormonal therapy;
3 radiation therapy;
4 open urinary diversion;
5 percutaneous urinary diversion; and
6 transurethral resection of the trigone with internal stenting.
Of these recently available treatment options it is the introduction of percutaneous urinary diversion that has been established as the initial diversion of choice, with an overall survival of 1 year (57%) and a median survival of 21 months if hormonal treatment has not already been given. These survival times are drastically reduced if the ureteric obstruction presents from a hormone resistant cancer either because of previous treatment or rarely a *de*

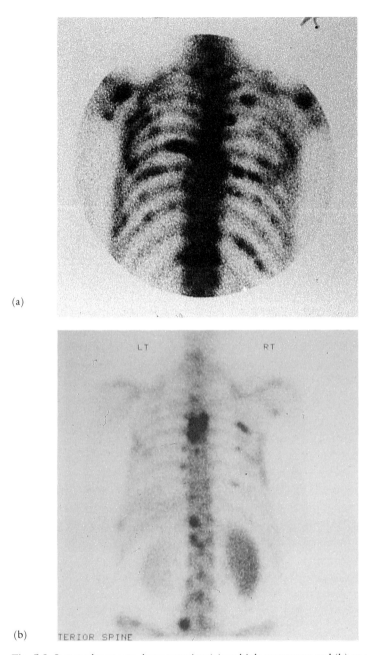

(a)

(b)

Fig. 5.1 Isotope bone scan demonstrating (a) multiple metastases and (b) an obstructed kidney, which was asymptomatic in this case.

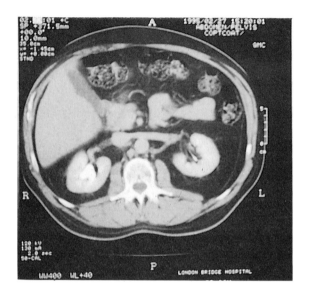

(a)

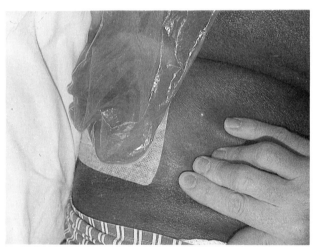

(b)

Fig. 5.2 (a) CT scan showing a right sided hydronephrosis secondary to paraortic lymphadenopathy caused by prostate cancer, a nephrostomy tube can be life saving but its subsequent management is difficult if hormone treatment has already failed. Most tubes need to be permanent and leak, requiring a stoma bag (b) and so we prefer to internally stent but this does require the use of double stents on both sides (Fig. 5.3).

novo characteristic. In these cases the mean survival of our own patients is only 5 months, with a range of 1–13 months.

A percutaneous urinary diversion can be carried out using local anaesthesia. It is usually performed in the radiology department but can be introduced on the ward under ultrasound control. Various manufactured sets are available for this procedure but the underlying principle is one of a hollow needle placement into the collecting system, preferably through the lower calyx. Direct puncture of the renal pelvis is a disadvantage because the subsequent stent is not held in place by the maximum amount of surrounding cortical tissue and is therefore prone to movement. A guide wire is fed in through the needle. A small vasal dilator is then passed over the guide wire (6 and 8 French); this allows for the relatively easy insertion of a 7 French nephrostomy tube into the collecting system. It is held to the skin surface by a stitch. The skin site is often a problem with long-term nephrostomy tubes where a chronic infection with granulation tissue can occur; this might need daily attention and dressing. This procedure is associated with minimal morbidity and no mortality in our series. The major complication is one of failure to gain access to an undilated connecting system (8%), significant haematuria which lasts for more than 24 hours (15%), and haemorrhage that requires a subsequent embolization (1%).

The nephrostomy tube can be supplanted by internal stenting in an antegrade fashion as retrograde attempts at inserting ureteric stents is usually unsuccessful due to invasion of the trigone and lower ureter. Again the results differ according to whether or not the patient has previously been treated with hormones. It is our policy to routinely replace a nephrostomy tube with an internal stent when the patient has only begun his first hormone treatment but in those hormone resistant cases, the replacement of a nephrostomy tube by a stent has worked in less then 10% of cases. This latter problem is due to the poor compliance of the ureter by either extensive peri-ureteric disease or involvement of the ureter itself (Fig. 5.3). One small practical point to remember is that if a ureteric stent is working well and the nephrostomy tube is temporarily left *in situ* as an insurance policy then there will be free reflux from the bladder to the stump drain of the nephrostomy tube. This is easily countered by the use of a urethral catheter until the nephrostomy tube is removed. Otherwise there is a danger of someone inadvertently thinking that the patient has experienced urinary retention.

The use of transurethral resection of a trigone invaded with cancer may sometimes facilitate the introduction of an internal stent particularly if the patient had a nephrostomy tube in place as precaution; methylene blue may

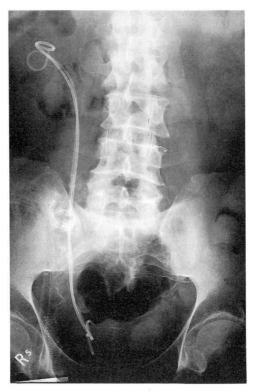

Fig. 5.3 An obstructive uropathy often cannot be temporized with a single ureteric stent because the poorly compliant malignant retroperitoneal tissue does not allow urine to pass around the stent. This can be overcome by the use of double stents, as shown in this X-ray. The first was inserted antegradely and the second at a subsequent cystoscopy.

be given intravenously to identify the lumen of the ureter once resection is completed. There is a certain danger of extravastion in these cases but we have been surprised at the low morbidity of this manoeuvre. Radiotherapy has been proposed as an alternative treatment but the results have been quite poor and those patients required diversion with or without internal stenting. It has been demonstrated that radiotherapy could increase the prostate size in 30% of cases (Carpenter & Schroder 1984). The results of open urinary diversion, whether as an open nephrostomy, cutaneous urethrostomy, or ileal conduit, have been consistently poor and it is certainly unfair to impose this type of surgery on a patient who may only have a few months to live. Fallon and colleagues (1980) reported a 49% post-operative complication rate and a 19% early mortality rate with an open urinary diversion in these cases, with an average hospital stay of up to 4 months.

Cancer pain

During the last 25 years, there has been a great upsurger of interest in the relief of cancer pain. This has been due in a large part to the modern hospice movement. She introduced two basic principles of pain control: the regular giving of analgesic drugs, and the titration of the dose against the patient's need. Since that time, further work has been done and the more specific causes of cancer pain have been studied. The place of adjuvant drug therapy has been clarified and the use of palliative radiotherapy has become more closely defined. Pain has been described as a psychosomatic experience with its intensity depending both on the extent of tissue damage and the patient's psychological state. The fear of physical deterioration, separation from family and ultimately death, will all exacerbate the perception of somatic sensations. Cancer pain is rarely an isolated physical symptom in a patient; anorexia, dyspnoea, nausea or vomiting, together with depression and anxiety, exacerbate the total pain experience.

The two most common sites affected by pain in prostate cancer patients are bone and less commonly, the perineum. A careful history of the pain is necessary; this should include the sites, severity and duration, aggravating and relieving factors, results of previous therapy and a verbatim description from the patient of their experience. The physical examination should note any motor or sensory changes or local tenderness, noting the possibility of referred pain. The psychological state of the patient and family should be assessed. A bone scan will be required to assess the overall spread of bone metastasis but plain X-rays will be required to assess particular painful sites and the associated risks of a pathological fracture Both computed tomography (CT) and magnetic resonance imaging (MRI) will confirm the local spread in the pelvis. It is tempting to attribute every pain in the cancer patient to his advancing malignant disease. However, in a study by Twycross (1993) no less than 33% of the pain in patients with advanced cancer was due to non-malignant causes related to treatment, debility or concurrent disease.

Principles of management

It goes without saying that treatment should be based on the accurate diagnosis of the cause of pain whenever possible, but sometimes the patient is confused or too ill for a full assessment to be made. In this situation analgesia must not be withheld. Mild pain can be treated with a non-opioid such as paracetamol, 1 g every 4 hours. If this is ineffective, the choice is between using a weak opioid such as codeine or a low dose of a strong opioid. This choice will depend on the expected rate of increase in severity of pain and the patient's prognosis. With escalating pain it is advisable to change directly from paracetamol to oral morphine.

Whatever analgesic is chosen it should be given regularly so that the therapeutic blood level is maintained throughout the 24 hours. There is no place for 'as required' analgesia in the constant pain of cancer. The dose interval would depend on the half-life of the drug and its active metabolites; this is the advantage of slow release morphine which has a half-life of 12 hours. One of the great advantages of morphine is the good correlation between dose and therapeutic effect within a wide range of doses. The majority of cancer patients are pain controlled on 30 mg MST (morphine sulphate tablets) twice daily.

Oral administration is preferred as it is more acceptable to the patient. The continuous subcutaneous infusion of a strong opioid may be required if there is vomiting, marked dyspnoea or coma. The place for spinal opioids in the management of severe cancer pain is not yet defined. Adjuvant drug therapy for pain control in cancer patients is important. Its use may mean that analgesics are not required at all, but more often the pain can be controlled with a lower dose of morphine. Non-steroidal anti-inflammatory drugs (NSAIDs) are used for pain from bone metastasis and they are occasionally helpful in pelvic pain. Corticosteroids reduce the inflammation around tumours and are particularly useful in the acute phase of a spinal cord compression; they have the added benefits of improving the well being of the patient. As anxiety and depression are known to exacerbate pain, their reduction will increase the pain relief obtained by other measures. A sympathetic explanation of the illness, good communication in the family, or even the resolution of financial or social problems, may have an analgesic affect. Anxiolytic or anti-depressant drugs may be required in addition to these measures. Palliative radiotherapy has an important role in the relief of pain from bone metastasis; it is less useful for pelvic pain caused by soft tissue infiltration.

Bone pain

This is the most common type of pain caused by prostate cancer and routine questioning of each patient is important because the symptoms are often insidious in onset and attributed to old age or arthritis. Such a self diagnosis may not actually be wrong, but it must not prevent the accurate diagnosis of the pain and help being offered. Eighty-five per cent of our patients with prostate cancer have bone metastases as shown on an isotope bone scan but only approximately half of these produce anything more than mild symptoms. The patients' description of the character of the pain is variable; different patients may use words which imply opposite characteristics such as dull/red-hot and aching/stabbing. An exacerbation with movement or pressure however is very common and pain on movement or tenderness over a bone suggests a metastasis until proven otherwise. A normal radiological appearance cannot exclude a bone metastasis and the isotopic scan is always seen as being more sensitive.

It is believed that prostacyclins are liberated by the majority of tumour deposits in bone (Lancet & Pezht 1975), causing both reabsorption of bone around the tumour and sensitization of nerve endings to painful stimuli. Bone metastases can therefore cause pain when they are very small. Treatment with NSAIDs is logical since they inhibit the synthesis of prostaglandins from arachidonic acid. As the metastases enlarge, they stretch the well innervated periosteum and eventually cause distortion of the bone under stress and may even lead to pathological fracture. Vertebral collapse may then lead to nerve root pain.

Treatment options

Radiotherapy must always be considered for these patients. Solitary metastases in long bones respond as well to single doses as to more prolonged courses, and a half body irradiation should be considered for widespread metastasis.

Radiotherapy

The application of radiotherapy for prostate cancer was pioneered in Europe by Paschkis (1910) who fixed a radium source to a cystoscope, and Pasteau (1913) who independently used a radium tube placed in an intra-urethral catheter. H.H. Young, who is more well known for his advocacy of surgery, took these ideas from Europe to the USA and began applying radium there in 1915. He used a variety of intra-urethral and intra-rectal radium sources as well as radium needles inserted into the prostate through the perineum, similar to contemporary techniques employed for implantation of the prostate with iodine-125. Palliative irradiation of patients with prostate cancer, largely for the relief of obstructive symptoms, was reported by Widmann (1934). Thereafter, radiotherapy gained a not unreasonable role as a treatment with curative intent.

Once definitive treatment for cure in the treatment of prostatic cancer is no longer an issue, palliation of regional symptomatology becomes a paramount concern. This is generally achieved, to a large degree but with a limited duration, by hormonal treatment. Radiation therapy may be used to relieve specific symptoms, both local and remote. It is usually required once hormonal treatment has begun to fail but may sometimes have a place early on in the management of a patient because hormonal treatment is very much relative in its effect and an individual patient may be left with a local site of pain. Relatively high doses of radiation must be utilized because the majority of prostate cancers are slow growing and require substantial radiation doses to provide significant regression. Because patients may also live for several years subsequently, even with significant local metastasis, irradiation must be carefully applied in order to minimize long-term radiation effects. Doses of about 40 Gy delivered over a period of 4 weeks (10 Gy/5-day week) are used. For symptoms secondary to urethral obstruction, doses of 50 or even 60 Gy may be required. These doses and fractionation patterns should produce a tumour regression without tissue injury. Single bone metastasis can usually be well palliated by doses of 40 Gy in 4 weeks at the rate of 2 Gy/day. Radiotherapy is much less helpful for lung, liver, brain or skin metastasis.

One very important indication for palliative irradiation is to prevent spinal cord compression. Areas of involvement in the vertebrae should be treated before structural damage threatens the integrity of the spinal cord. Its radiation dose must be relatively high in order to stop the progression, between 40 and 50 Gy delivered at the rate of 2 Gy/day is required.

Hemibody irradiation

Focal irradiation is certainly effective in palliating bony pain. However it is not unusual for multiple sites of bone metastasis to become symptomatic simultaneously or within a short interval. If each site is radiated singularly, the patient may be inconvenienced by several weeks of treatment in succession. Therefore hemibody irradiation is a logical alternative for providing patients who have disseminated prostate cancer with symptomatic relief in the least inconvenient manner. Fitzpatrick & Rider (1976) began a programme of wide field irradiation, treating patients with advanced and symptomatic prostate cancer refractory to other treatment methods. The field and dose were gradually increased so that finally, 1000 cGy was delivered to a half body. Some patients' symptoms were so severe that after appropriate marrow recovery, the other half of the body was treated as well.

The entire body is not treated simultaneously because the dose that can be applied safely to the whole body is much lower than that which can be delivered to either half. The dose for total body irradiation may not exceed 300 cGY in either single or fractionated doses because of the risk of lethal bone marrow toxicity. Therefore, although total body irradiation has been employed effectively in the treatment of haematology malignancies which typically are very radio-sensitive, it would not be beneficial for most solid tumours.

Van de Werf Messing applied selective sequential hemibody irradiation to patients with prostate cancer who had lymph node involvement or high grade tumours and were therefore at risk of developing disease dissemination (Rubin *et al.* 1985). Compared to historical controls, patients treated in this manner appear to have about a one and a half year delay in the appearance of distal metastasis. There was also improvement in metastasis-free survival. However, these early encouraging results have not been reproduced and any positive effect was unfortunately lost in patient selection.

Hemibody irradiation remains an excellent tool but in a palliative context only. Although it does not always require hospitalization as acute side effects can be managed quite well with adequate premedication, short overnight stay is often employed, especially in the more debilitated patients and for upper half body therapy. The typical pre-treatment regimen for upper half body irradiation includes intravenous fluids, antiemetic drugs and corticosteroids. Antiemetics are also routinely administered prior to lower half body treatment. The upper and lower half fields are shown in Fig. 5.4. The upper half body field typically extends from above the scalp to the umbilicus at the level of the iliac crest, and the lower half body field from the umbilicus to the ankles. The eyes, mouth and thyroid gland can be shielded, and with upper half body doses greater than 600 cGY, partial transmission lung blocks are recommended to avoid unnecessary pulmonary toxicity. In patients previously irradiated, a spinal cord block may also be necessary to avoid exceeding organ tolerance. Because of extended distances, up to 30 minutes treatment time is typically required, in contrast to the very short treatment times of focal irradiation treatment. After 4–6 weeks, when blood counts have returned to their baseline level, patients can be considered for treatment to the other hemibody field if symptoms in that area demand it.

Tumour responses in terms of measured regression is not frequently reported, but pain relief is very effective. Complete pain relief has been reported in 24–70% of patients and partial relief of pain in 24–71% (Pene 1981; Reed *et al.* 1988). The average time course of response to hemibody

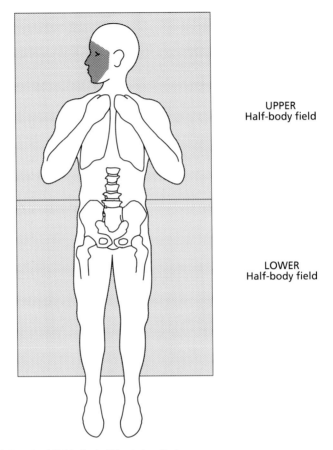

UPPER
Half-body field

LOWER
Half-body field

Fig. 5.4 Standard fields for half body irradiation.

irradiation unfortunately only approximates 6 months but it does not preclude additional use of localized treatment to areas of recurrence or new symptoms. Such a timescale often represents the majority of the patient's remaining life; therefore there is gratitude that this is a relatively pain-free period since most of these patients will also have become hormone resistant, and other adjunctive forms of systemic treatment may become progressively unpleasant in the debilitated patient.

The acute side effects of hemibody irradiation are defined as those occurring immediately after and up to 2 weeks after treatment. Acute radiation syndrome is seen within 1–2 hours and subsides within 8–10 hours. It is similar to a stress reaction caused by a lack of adrenal reserve, and although it is significant with upper body irradiation, it is mild or absent with lower half body therapy. The symptoms include nausea, vomiting, increase in temperature and pulse rate and hypotension; these can be minimized by the pre-medication indicated above. These side effects normally resolve within 24 hours. Diarrhoea can present in up to 75% of cases of lower field treatment usually beginning 2–3 days after therapy. Again this usually subsides shortly afterwards but pre-medication is again helpful.

The two most life threatening effects are bone marrow toxicity and radiation pneumonia. Bone marrow toxicity occurs to a large extent in up to 25% of patients and in 10% the effects are potentially life threatening but rarely fatal. These effects are exaggerated if the patient has received previous thermotherapy as they may have a compromised marrow before treatment. Weekly blood counts are recommended in the presence of a severe neutropenia and symptoms of infection. Then, broad spectrum antibiotics must be used immediately together with reversed barrier nursing. Such patients are very vulnerable. The marrow should return to normal over a period of 4–6 weeks. Several authors have reported a significant incidence of radiation pneumonitis which proved fatal in over 65% of patients (Keen 1980). This complication was found to be dose-related and the incidence dropped remarkably with dose reduction. The symptoms of cough and dyspnoea occur between 30 and 120 days after treatment.

Other less significant subacute effects of hemibody irradiation include stomatitis, conjunctivitis, pharyngitis, oesophagitis and alopecia, some of which can be avoided by blocking the mouth, eyes and thyroid gland. After over 30 years experience of hemibody irradiation, the consensus of opinion is that a dose of 600 cGy for the upper half and 800 cGy for the lower half of the body are the safest and the most effective doses tested with the possibility of maximum pain relief and minimum side effects. Evaluation of hemibody irradiation certainly shows this to be much more life threatening than simple hormonal treatment, but it must be borne in mind that the vast majority of patients for whom this is indicated have already become resistant to hormone manipulation and the alternative may be a short life of poor quality on high doses of opioid analgesics. An alternative radiotherapy tool also indicated in patients with widespread, painful bone metastases, is the use of intravenous strontium, but the experience with this is much shorter and the side effects much less predictable. Strontium treatment however, does have the great advantage that it can be given in a smaller hospital with nuclear medicine facilities that may not have easy access to a linear accelerator.

Radio-pharmaceuticals for bone pain

Hemibody radiation is useful in patients with diffused or rapidly recurring pain but it is accompanied by significant toxicity and is therefore difficult to use as a repeatable treatment. There is need for an effective, well tolerated systemic therapy that can be repeated and this is the objective of a radio-pharmaceutical. It is a form of systemic radiotherapy *in situ* where the radio-pharmaceutical is concentrated at the site of the metastatic lesion. This approach is not entirely new and over recent years many agents have been tested. However, the success of various nuclides used have been variable (Ketering *et al.* 1986). More recently, strontium-89 chloride (Metastron) has undergone extensive clinician trials. It is a more specific mode of action leading to an efficient localization at the site of a bone metastases. Through selective beta radiation of multiple sites simultaneously, it has provided pain relief for an average period of up to 6 months in up to 80% of patients with hormone resistant bone pain whilst causing minor haematological side effects (Robinson 1987). It has also been used at an earlier stage in the disease process before the onset of bone pain in patients with a partial resolution of bone metastasis seen on bone scans (Porter & Chisholm 1993), and is a reasonable alternative to external beam irradiation when the latter is not easily and readily available.

Strontium-89 imitates the *in vivo* behaviour of calcium and is preferentially taken up by bone. It concentrates at sites of high metabolism such as osteoblastic metastasis and is washed out of healthy bone. Strontium-89 has a biological half-life of approximately 14 days in normal bone, but in bone affected by metastasis the retention is extremely prolonged. It is primarily excreted by the kidney and so caution is necessary in patients with renal impairment. The uptake and retention of strontium in patients with bone metastasis has been investigated with the radiotracer strontium-85 which mimics the behaviour of strontium-89; because it has gamma omission, it is convenient for measurement. Patients with varying volumes of metastatic disease will clear the isotope at varying rates. Whole body retention can vary between 11% in those with minimal volume disease to 88% in a patient with complete skeletal involvement. This can carry distinct disadvantages for a patient who may then experience a delayed marrow suppression and an associated anaemia and vulnerability to infection. A full blood count must be carried out at least weekly for 4 weeks following treatment.

Pathological fractures

Pathological fractures are of two kinds: those occurring in apparently normal bone (stress fractures), and those occurring in bone which is abnormal. Metastatic prostate cancer deposits weaken bone and predispose it to pathological fracture. The most commonly affected sites are the spine, femur (neck and shaft), humerus and pelvis. Ninety per cent of prostate cancer bone deposits are osteosclerotic, due to an increase in local osteo-blastic activity. This might give the impression of an overcalcified and perhaps invulnerable site, but this is not the case. There may be an increased localized mineral content but the bone architecture is abnormal and unable to bear extreme forces of compression.

A patient with a pathological fracture usually presents as an emergency to the orthopaedic department. It has become an infrequent 'first' pre-sentation of prostate cancer in the last decade, presumably because of earlier referral and investigations of prostatic symptoms. A plain X-ray of a long bone fracture will demonstrate a cortex thinned or eroded by the deposit, and usually a medulla with an increased density. A plain X-ray of a patho-logical vertebral crush fracture is a little more difficult to distinguish from a benign form. It is usually associated with a history of only a mild stress injury such as jumping from a single step. An ordinary crush fracture is nearly always of the upper border. With a fracture through malignant disease, the anterior border may be eroded. Orthopaedic surgeons are not accustomed to carrying out a rectal examination but this will often clinch the diagnosis. It should be confirmed with a prostate biopsy, serum prostate specific antigen (PSA) measurement and a whole body radionuclide scan.

A metastatic deposit is not the only cause for a pathological fracture in a patient with advanced prostate cancer. Long term use of a luteinizing hormone-releasing hormone (LHRH) analogue can produce a subclinical loss of bone calcium, so much so that some clinicians advocate the use of regular scans and calcium supplements. Obvious clinical osteoporosis is rare, but all patients will have a slightly increased susceptibility to a stress fracture of the femoral neck. A femoral neck fracture is treated by internal fixation, but a bone biopsy may be needed at the time of operation to exclude a metastatic deposit that may have been assumed because of the patient's primary diagnosis. This will have relevance in choosing between the need for future calcium supplements or possibly adjuvant radiotherapy.

Pathological fractures due to metastatic deposits may unite with con-servative treatment, especially with adjuvant radiotherapy and hormonal treatment if not already used. Internal fixation (Fig. 5.5) is, however, often

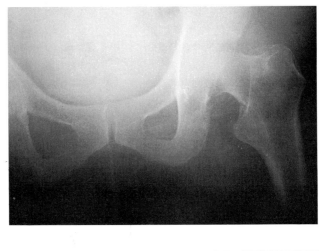

(a)

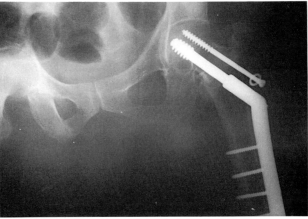

(b)

Fig. 5.5 (a) Pathological fracture of the neck of the left femur. (b) Fractures such as these, through secondary deposits, are nearly always treated by internal fixation.

preferred because it enables the patient to enjoy activity during his remaining months of life. If the bone is too weak for the metal to hold securely, one answer is to pack the bone interior with acrylic cement before plating.

Just as close supervision of prostate cancer patients with increasing back pain is required to avoid spinal cord compression by the early use of radiotherapy, so is there a need to be alert to the patient and pain in a weight bearing bone. Early assessment of a bone deposit will allow prompt radiotherapy which is not only palliative with regard to pain, but will also facilitate partial regrowth of normal bone architecture, in doing so avoiding a pathological fracture. Internal fixation is also recommended as a pre-ventative measure if more than 50% of the cortex has been eroded. In these cases radiotherapy alone is not sufficient.

Spinal cord compression

The treatment of spinal cord compression secondary to metastatic prostate cancer is palliative. An important goal is to prevent the condition. It is a sad fact to relate that of the 14 cases of cord compression that presented to our department in the last 3 years, nine of them had sought medical advice in the preceding weeks, complaining of increasing back pain; these were all patients with known prostate cancer. All medical practitioners must be aware that a patient with advanced prostate cancer, with new or changing symptoms of back pain, must be assessed immediately with at least an iso-tope bone scan and plain X-ray, but ideally also with an MRI scan (Fig. 5.6). Missed cases such as these will rarely regain normal function, even with intensive treatment. Prevention cannot be a point exaggerated enough. A patient paralysed from spinal cord compression may live for many months with frequent problems associated with bladder catheter-ization, pressure sores and infections. This justifies aggressive treatment to attempt to reverse cord compression and prompt action is the key. The site of involvement is usually in the thoracic spine (60%) and can involve the cauda equina (40%). Patients with these conditions are managed in a similar way.

Approximately 5% of prostate cancer patients develop extradural tumour deposits (Black 1979), but we have seen a dramatic increase in this figure since the introduction of maximum androgen blockade (MAB). The number of patients presenting with spinal cord compression has dramati-cally risen from a mean of approximately 4% per year in the last decade, to 14% per year in the last 5 years. This may simply reflect a change in referral patterns where the patients were previously sent to either the neurosurgical unit or admitted directly to a hospice for terminal care. Alternatively it could represent the natural selection of hormonal resistant cancers in patients with an increased survival because of the early introduction of MAB to patients with a low volume disease. In metastatic prostate cancer the extradural (epidural) space of a spinal cord is involved secondarily by extension from an eroded vertebral body arch or spinal process. There must also be an element of compression secondary to the collapse or displacement of a bony ele-ment. Direct tumour extension is however the most common mechanism of extrinsic compression. Significant vertebral body collapse, especially with

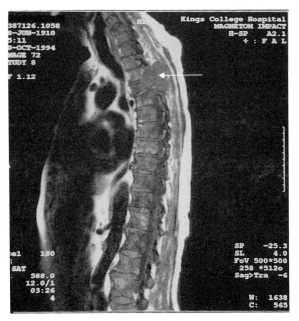

Fig. 5.6 This T2-weighted MRI scan shows the site of spinal cord compression in the thoracic spine.

angulation of the spine, appears to make the prognosis for recovery less favourable. Most often the cancer extends from an anterior eroded vertebral body posteriorly to compress the dura which in turn compresses the cord. The tumour compresses the blood supply of the cord from the epidural space, with the dura being an effective barrier to penetration. Intradural metastases are rare. The main signs and symptoms that characterize spinal cord or cauda equina compression are pain, weakness, autonomic dysfunction and sensory loss. Pain is an initial symptom in more than 90% of patients and is usually present from days to months before the diagnosis is established, although the major neurological deficit is sometimes quite spectacularly associated with a sudden pain representing acute vertebral collapse. This can often be provoked by simple acts such as coming down a step or even coughing. Fortunately, many prostatic cancer patients with back pain secondary to spinal metastatic disease never develop clinically evident cord compression as they are often treated with radiation or endocrine therapy for symptomatic bone metastasis prior to its development.

Previously, myelography was essential for the diagnosis of spinal cord compression. This was a difficult and sometimes painful procedure. MRI has now become the primary radiological procedure for the diagnosis and very accurate localization of cord compression. It is less invasive and better tolerated than myelography. MRI also has the ability to demonstrate both osteolytic and osteoblastic metastases and it has been a surprise to us that up to 10% of spinal metastases in our patients have proved to be osteolytic. Analysis of patients presenting with spinal cord compression in our own department has shown that 10% also presented with more than one site of potential compression.

Palliation is the goal of treatment but this should not prevent prompt evaluation and action. There is a strong correlation between pre-treatment motor status and treatment outcome, but this under scores the importance of prompt treatment before further neurological deterioration occurs: before damage to the spinal cord becomes permanent. High dose steroids (dexamethasone) should be instituted immediately, and hormonal treatment should be started, if not already in use. Ambulatory and moderately paraplegic patients seem best treated initially with radiation alone. Immediate surgical decompression should be used in patients with an expected life span of at least 6 months who deteriorate during radiation, who have had previous irradiation to the involved site, or who have a potentially correctable and stable spine.

Hormonal treatment has always had a prominent role in the treatment of spinal cord compression in the newly presenting patient. But this is now rare: only one patient in the last 5 years has presented in this way to our department and benefited from hormonal treatment. The remaining patients have all presented with hormone resistant prostate cancer as judged by a rising PSA whilst on hormonal treatment. Definitive treatment of spinal cord compression is brought about by the use of radiation, surgery or a combination of both. In a series of patients treated primarily by surgery, Shoskes & Perrin (1989) reported that all 15 ambulatory patients remained ambulatory and 8 out of 13 bed-ridden patients (62%) became ambulatory post-operatively. In a similar surgical series, all seven ambulatory patients remained ambulatory and 14 of 27 bed-ridden patients (52%) became ambulatory post-operatively. In that series, of the 20 patients who could walk after a decompression laminectomy, 15 remained ambulatory until death. Of the 18 patients who required urinary catheterization, nine made sufficient recovery to make this unnecessary. Of the entire group of 34 patients who complained of back pain, decompression relieved pain in 26 (77%), sufficiently to stop the narcotic analgesics. Such surgery however is not without risk and in the latter series, there was a peri-operative death rate of 8%. The best success with treatment by radiation alone is with ambulatory and moderately paraparetic patients, not with paraplegic patients in whom the results are poor (Barcena 1984).

The overall survival after the diagnosis of spinal cord compression from epidural metastatic prostate cancer would depend greatly on whether the patient has hormone resistant cancer. In these cases, survival may be of no more than 12 months with a mean of 6 months. Patients who receive immediate surgery or radiation and are commenced on hormone treatment as a combined primary form of management, have a relatively good survival with a mean duration of 16 months. Early attention to patients with known metastatic prostate cancer and increasing back pain cannot be exaggerated. Treatment of back pain with either focal radiotherapy or hemibody irradiation will prevent the majority of spinal cord compression cases developing to a clinical level. Spinal cord compression, when it does develop, must be assessed by MRI and treated promptly. It is sometimes very difficult to interest a neurosurgeon in a case which at beast may seem to deserve only palliative treatment. However surgical intervention in patients who present with paraplegia, or who develop the paraplegia during assessment, carries the best chance of a return to normal neurological function. This in turn will improve the quality of the patient's life in their remaining days and make the nursing care of this patient far easier.

Pelvic pain

Pelvic pain can be caused by widespread metastasis in the bony pelvis and this will be obvious on both a bone scan and play X-ray. Pelvic pain can also be caused by local spread of the tumour. Such pain is most commonly felt in the rectum. Phrases used to describe this rectal pain fall into two groups: rectal fullness and severe shooting pain. The perineum and genitalia are occasional sites of referred pain. Pain is sometimes made worse by sitting down or by constipation. New strong opioids are the mainstay of treatment. Simple, local procedures are frequently helpful. These include faecal disimpaction, catheterization, steroid retention enemas; nerve blocks should be considered with tractable pelvic pain. The two most useful procedures are a lumbar intra-thecal block for perineal and genital pain, and a lumbar sympathetic block for tenesmus and phantom rectal pain. Palliative radiotherapy can sometimes help by reducing pressure but there is a risk of fissure formation, especially in previously irradiated patients.

Hypercalcaemia

Much of the bone destruction in metastasis is mediated not by the tumour cell but by the patient's normal osteoclasts. This increased osteoclastic activity is readily detected biochemically by a raised alkaline phosphatase. Biphosphonates are analogues of pyrophosphates (POP) in which the POP backbone is replaced by a form that is more resistant to enzymatic hydrolysis. The role of biphosphonates in the treatment of malignant hypercalcaemia is now well established, and recent randomized trials have shown a reduction in the complications of bone metastasis following adjuvant clodronate treatment for both myeloma and breast cancer. Benefits reported included a reduction in pain and hence less need for analgesics and radiotherapy. A reduction in the incidence of hypercalcaemia and pathological fractures have also been reported. Clodronate has also been shown to reduce increased bone resorption due to malignancy in the absence of hypercalcaemia (Adami & Mian 1989).

Holistic requirements

Holism is the consideration of the complete person in the treatment of their disease. It raises the importance of the psychological well being of the patient at the time of diagnosis, and for many, during a terminal illness. In 1990 the World Health Organization (WHO) adopted a definition of palliative care as the 'total active care of patients whose disease is not responsive to curative treatment and that the control of pain, other symptoms and psychological, social and spiritual problems is paramount'. A sense of peace and well being is not a natural reaction for the majority of men, but there is both physical and psychological support that can be titrated to great effect. The most significant single problem is anxiety. The temperance of anxiety by communication and trust cannot be underestimated. Of the advances in cancer care that have evolved in the last decade I rank the honest counselling of a cancer patient and his family to be at the forefront. This has been extended to a patient's grandchildren so that a happy grandfather can even be surrounded by his whole family during his terminal illness, even if this is in a hospice. These advances will only be seen if the care is holistic and the surgeon and oncologist work closely with cancer counsellors and palliative care workers. The ideal palliative care team should have as its members: a doctor, a nurse, a pharmacist, a physiotherapist, an occupational therapist, a dietician, a MacMillan nurse, a social worker, a chaplain, a counsellor and an incontinence advisor. These are the foundations of quality cancer care that should be present in every hospital and far surpass the value of hi-tech equipment, surgeons or molecular therapy.

There is a traditional view amongst both patients and doctors that prostate cancer is part and parcel of old age and that one has to die of something sometime, so why not prostate cancer? This is in contrast to the perception of cancer in the younger female population which has led to intense lobbying and the quite legitimate introduction of early screening programmes for cervical, breast and now ovarian cancers. The male elderly population is realizing that its life expectancy and the quality of that life, is now superior. In line with this is the general feeling that patients do not want to die from prostate cancer, nor suffer the complications of prostate cancer if these can be avoided. Whilst we have not yet seen an intense lobbying campaign from this group for better screening programmes, there is at least an atmosphere where free and open communication on these issues is pertinent and important.

We have established a policy of optimum communication with the patient at all stages of their disease process. This even includes informed consent for a PSA examination. It is quite clear that there is little time for important matters concerning the patient's diagnosis, his expectations, his family's fears and some idea of a prognosis in a busy outpatient clinic. We have begun a specialized prostate cancer clinic in which there is not only more time to counsel each patient, but there is also a palliative care nurse present. The role of palliative care starts with the diagnosis of prostate cancer and should not be reserved for the terminally ill.

In order to reinforce the concept of counselling and early support, we have begun a policy of giving the patients a copy of their own prostate cancer record similar to that used in obstetrics. This is most important for follow-up, where each symptom is scored as well as the accepted parameters of the disease. An indication is also given as to the patient's current understanding of their disease and this has led to a far greater under- standing, especially from the associated family. A small spin-off has also been that the patient's hospital records do not need to be at hand at that the patient can also take his current treatment record along to either his family practitioner, or any doctor that he may need to see whilst away from his locality.

Complementary medicine has also probably been under-used in the past because it was seen to have its main role in the terminally ill when more established treatments had failed. This is again unfair for the majority of patients who could benefit from various aspects of complementary medicine if this was offered as soon as the diagnosis was made. Both massage and aromatherapy are offered to our patients at every stage of their illness. An active patient awaiting a curative radical prostatectomy and a bed-bound patient receiving parenteral morphine may both find their anxieties softened by these therapies. Herbal remedies have no unique role in the treatment of prostate cancer, but I do routinely prescribe Iscador (mistletoe extract) and Lycopodium to patients with hormone refractory disease. Iscador produces a mild granulocytosis with a possible enhancement of the immune system and Lycopodium is a constitutional prescription. There is no scientific data to support their use and perhaps it is the psychological support that comes with the more holistic nature of those that prescribe them that benefits most patients. Anyone who has sat in an oncology clinic at the London Homeopathic Hospital will have been impressed with the sense of well being and peace in all the patients.

If they wish, whenever possible, patients should be allowed to die in their own homes. Although families may at first be afraid of caring for the patient at home, they will usually do so if extra support from district nursing services is provided. Families may be reassured if an assurance is given that the patient will be admitted to a hospital or hospice if they cannot cope. The role of the hospice has changed: with the centralization of specialized cancer centres, the hospice is often becoming a community focus of cancer treatment and palliative care. Thank goodness the days have gone when a patient's only valid ticket of entry into a hospice was one way and with a predicted stay of less than 6 months.

There is a temptation to finish this chapter with a list of miscellaneous cancer related problems and their remedies, but an inability to find a suitable heading should not diminish their importance. They are the very issues which may make a difference in quality during the patient's last weeks of life and are essential facets of holistic care.

Intractable pain

The routine use of oral analgesics has been described above. However there sometimes comes a point when breakthrough pain occurs even when using oral morphine. Modified-release tablets are an alternative to the oral solution; they have a longer action and need only be taken every 12 hours. When replacing a weaker opioid analgesic, the starting dose is usually 20–30 mg twice daily. Increments should be made to the dose not the frequency of administration. If the patient becomes unable to swallow, the equivalent intramuscular dose of morphine is half the oral solution dose; in the case of the modified-release tablets it is half the 24-hour dose (which is then divided into six portions to be given every 4 hours). Diamorphine is preferred for injection because, being more soluble, it can be given in a smaller volume. Repeated injections into a cachexic patient are unfair and a more reasonable parenteral method is a continuous subcutaneous infusion given by a syringe driver. The equivalent doses of morphine (oral and MST) and diamorphine are shown in Table 5.1. The general principle that injections should be given into separate sites and should not be mixed does not apply to syringe drivers in terminal care. Provided that there is evidence of compatibility, selected injections can be mixed in syringe drivers. In particular, chlorpromazine and diazepam are contraindicated because they cause skin reactions at the injection site. The equivalent continuous dose of diamorphine is shown in Table 5.1. The following drugs can be mixed with diamorphine: cyclizine, dexamethazone, haloperidol, metoclopramide and midazolam. If breakthrough pain occurs during a continuous infusion then a subcutaneous (preferably) or intramuscular injection of diamorphine equivalent to one-sixth of the total 24-hour subcutaneous infusion is given. It is better to give this as an intermittent bolus injection via a subcutaneous butterfly needle. To minimize the risk of infection, no individual sub-cutaneous infusions should be used for longer than 24 hours.

Table 5.1 The equivalent doses of morphine (oral and MST) and diamorphine required for pain relief in advanced prostate cancer. These doses are approximate and may need to be adjusted according to response.

Oral morphine (mg)		Parenteral diamorphine (mg)	
Morphine sulphate oral solution or standard tablets (Every 4 hours)	Morphine sulphate modified-release tablets (Every 12 hours)	Diamorphine hydrochloride by intramuscular injection (Every 4 hours)	Diamorphine hydrochloride by subcutaneous infusion (Every 24 hours)
5	20	2.5	15
10	30	5	20
15	50	5	30
20	60	7.5	45
30	90	10	60
40	120	15	90
60	180	20	120
80	240	30	180
100	300	40	240
130	400	50	300
160	500	60	360
200	600	70	400

Anorexia and malaise

Anorexia may be helped by prednisolone 15–30 mg daily. A general feeling of malaise and tiredness may also be temporized in this way, but anaemia must be excluded. Marrow replacement by metastatic disease, or suppression caused by radiotherapy or radiopharmaceuticals may require repeated transfusions. This is an excellent role for a hospice where a short stay for a transfusion can make life at home much more reasonable.

Constipation

Constipation is a very common cause of distress and is almost invariable after administration of an opioid. It should be prevented if possible by the regular administration of laxatives. Lactulose solution with a senna preparation can be used.

Oral candidiasis

A dry mouth can be a side effect of diamorphine but it may also be associated with candidiasis, especially if the patient has recently been on a broad-spectrum antibiotic and chemotherapy. It has the typical appearance of white plaques on the tongue that bleed on manipulation (Fig. 5.7). It can be treated by nystatin oral suspension or amphotericin lozenges. Persistent oral candidiasis, in the presence of a suppressed immune system will require intravenous fluconazole. This is also needed for oesophageal candidiasis which is not uncommon, should be suspected when the symptoms of dysphagia are out of proportion to the oral signs, and does not require the patient to go through an unpleasant oesophagoscopy to prove the diagnosis.

Nausea and vomiting

Nausea and vomiting may occur in the initial stages of morphine therapy but can be prevented by giving an antiemetic such as haloperidol or prochlorperazine. An antiemetic is usually only necessary for the first 4–5 days. Their further routine use may lead to unnecessary drowsiness. An antiemetic can be given in a syringe driver.

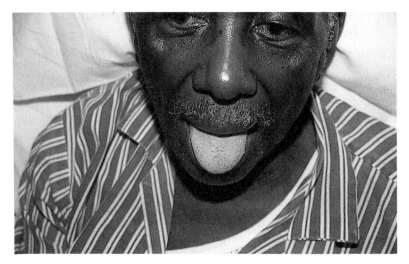

Fig. 5.7 The typical appearances of oral candidiasis and vitamin deficiency in a patient with advanced hormone resistant cancer who has been on oral chemotherapy for 3 weeks. There is a great danger of opportunistic infections in these immunosuppressed patients. The net gain is negligible except that everyone feels that 'something is being done'.

Insomnia

Patients with advanced cancer may not sleep because of discomfort, cramps, night sweats, joint stiffness or fear. There should be appropriate treatment of these problems before hypnotics are used. Benzodiazepines such as temazepam may be useful, but often in a friendly environment such as their home, or even a hospice, a warm milk drink or a glass of stout is preferred.

It is quite apparent that many of these problems that bedevil a terminally ill patient are the result of a perhaps unrealistic belief that we can dramatically alter the destiny of that patient. Faced with the reality of a malignant disease, many patients (and their relatives) will be prepared to accept a treatment of high toxicity for even a small chance of benefit (Slevin 1990). We are the gate-keepers of treatment regimens that may not prolong survival and yet produce a complex interaction of complications that make the important last days of a patient unnecessarily unpleasant. We have a responsibility to recognize the quality and value of an individual's life whilst not withholding information or treatment that a patient may choose to have.

Practice points

- Ureteric obstruction will often respond to hormonal treatment if not previously used, and temporising nephrostomy diversion can be life saving.
- Ureteric obstruction in a patient with hormone resistant disease is a difficult management problem. A reasonable palliative treatment is initial nephrostomy tube insertion, followed by antegrade ureteric stenting; double stenting on each side is essential because of impaired ureteric wall compliance.
- Pain can be palliated with local or hemibody irradiation. Radio-pharmaceuticals have the advantage of short-term success and can be repeated, but are associated with marrow suppression and should be used with caution.
- A negative bone scan in a patient on hormonal treatment merely indicates quiescence of osteoblastic activity and may hide a silent metastasis. A MRI scan is essential to exclude incipient spinal cord compression when there is back pain.
- Early treatment of spinal cord compression is essential if neurological sequelae are to be minimized. The majority of these patients have hormone resistant disease. Local radiotherapy is successful when signs are mild but severe neurological impairment warrants an urgent neurosurgical opinion.
- The final months of a patients life can be transformed by an holistic and team approach. Attention to anxiety and peripheral medical problems will allow a patient to die with dignity.

References

Adami, Mian M. (1989) Clodronate therapy of metastatic bone disease in patients with prostatic carcinoma. *Recent Results Can. Res.*, **116**, 67–72.

Adamson A.S., Francis J.L., Witherow R.O., Snell M.E. (1994) Procoagulant properties of benign and malignant prostatic tissue. *Br. J. Urol.*, **74**(2), 204–209.

Addonizio J.C. (1982) Another look at cryoprostatectomy. *Cryobiology*, **19**, 223–227.

Akakura K., Bruchovsky N., Goldenberg S.L., Rennie P.S., Buckley A.R., Sullivan L.D. (1993) Effects of intermittent androgen suppression on androgen-dependent tumours. Apoptosis and serum prostate-specific antigen. *Cancer*, **71**, 2782–2790.

Albarran, Halle N. (1900) Hypertrophie et neoplasies epitherliales de la prostate. *Ann. Nial. Org. Gen. Urin.*, **18**, 113 & 225.

Aprikian M., Bazinet M., Plaute A. *et al.* (1995) Family history and risk of prostatic carcinoma in high risk groups of urological patients. *J. Urol.*, **154**, 404–406.

Avs G., Hugusson J., Norlen L. (1995) Need for hospital care and palliative treatment for prostate cancer treated with non-curative intent. *J. Urol.*, **154**, 466–469.

Bandhauer K. (1975) The possible role of transurethral resection in the dissemination of prostate cancer. *Euro. Urol.*, **1**, 272–274.

Barcena A., Lobato R.D., Rivas J.J. *et al.* (1984) Spinal metastatic disease: An analysis of factors determining functional prognosis and the choice of treatment. *Neurosurgery*, **15**, 820–827.

Baron J. (1940) Roentgenologic observation of formation of calcium carbonate gall-stone. *Radiology*, **35**, 741–742.

Black P. (1979) Spinal metastasis: current status and recommended guidelines for management. *Neurosurgery*, **5**, 726–746.

Blackard C.E., Byar D.P. (1972) Results of a clinical trial of surgery and radiation in stages ii and 3 carcinoma of the bladder. *J. Urol.*, **108**, 875–878.

Bonney W.W., Henstorf J.E., Emasus S.P., Lubaroff D.M., Feldbush T.L. (1978) Immunosuppression by cryosurgery: an orthotopic model of prostate and bladder cancer in the rat. *Natl. Cancer Inst. Monogr.*, **49**, 375–381.

Bostwick (1995) *National History of Early Prostate Cancer.* ICI, Proceedings of a Paris Meeting.

Bracci U. (1979) Antiandrogens in the treatment of prostatic cancer. *Eur. Urol.*, **5**, 303.

Brodie B.C. (1849) *Lectures on Diseases of Urinary Organs*, 4th edition. Green, Brown and Longman, London.

Byar D.P. (1972) Survival of patients with incidentally found microscopic cancer of the prostate; results of a clinical trial of conservative treatment. *J. Urol*, **108**, 908–913.

Byar D.P. (1977) (Editorial) Sound advice for conducting clinical trials. *N. Engl. J. Med.*, **297** (10), 553–554.

Carpenter B.J., Schroder F.H. (1984) Transrectal ultrasound of prostatic carcinoma patients; a new prognostic parameter? *J. Urol.*, **131**(5), 903–905.

Casper R.F., Yen S.S. (1985) Neuroendocrinology of menopausal flushes; an hypothesis of flush mechanism. *Clin. Endocrin. (Oxf.)*, **22**(3), 293–312.

Cassileth B.R., Soloway M.S., Vogellang N.J. *et al.* (1989) Patients choice of treatment in stage D prostate cancer. *Urology*, **33**(Suppl. 5), 57–62.

Chadwick D.J. *et al.* (1991) Comparison of TRUS and MRI in staging prostate cancer. *Br. J. Urol.*, **67**, 616–621.

Chisholm G.D. (1990) Chemotherapy for prostate cancer. Present concerns and future considerations. *Drugs*, **39**(3), 331–336.

Chlebowski J.F., Mabrey S. (1977) Differential scanning calorimetry of apro-, apophosphoryl and metalloalkaline phosphatases. *J. Biol. Chem.*, **252**(2), 7042–7052.

Chlebowski J.F., Armitage I.M., Coleman J.E. (1977) Allosteric interactions between metal ion and phosphate at the active sites of alkaline phosphatase as determined by ^{31}P-NMR and ^{113}Cd-NMR. *J. Biol. Chem.*, **252**(20), 7053–7061.

Chlebowski R.T., Herstorff R., Sardoff L., Weiner J., Bateman J.R. (1978) Cyclophosphamide versus the combination of adriamycin, 5-flurouracil and cyclophosphamide in the treatment of metastatic prostate cancer. A randomised trial. *Cancer*, **42**, 2546–2552.

Christensson A., Bjork T., Nilsson O. *et al.* (1993) Serum prostate specific antigen complexed to alpha 1-antichymotrypsin as an indicator of prostate cancer. *J. Urol.*, **150**(1), 100–105.

Chybowski F.M., Keller J.J., Bergstralh E.J., Oesterling J.E. (1991) Predicting radionuclide bone scan findings in patients with newly diagnosed untreated prostatic cancer: prostate specific antigen is superior to all other clinical parameters. *J. Urol.*, **145**(2), 313–318.

Civantos F., Marcial M.A., Banks E.R. *et al.* (1995) Pathology of androgen deprivation therapy in prostate carcinoma. *Cancer*, **75**(7), 1634–1641.

Clegg E.J. (1955) The arterial supply of the human prostate and seminal vesicles. *J. Anat.*, **89**, 209–216.

Coffey D.S., Pienta K.J. (1987) New concepts in studying the control of normal and cancer growth of the prostate. *Prog. Clin. Biol. Res.*, **239**, 1.

Cooner W.H., Mosley B.R., Rutherford C.L. Jr. *et al.* (1990) Prostate cancer detection in a clinical urological practice by ultrasonography, digital rectal examination and prostate specific antigen. *J. Urol.*, **143**(6), 1146–1152. (Discussion 1152–1154).

Cooper E.H., Siddall J.K., Newling D.W., Robinson M.R. (1988) Acid phosphate, alkaline phosphatase and prostate specific antigen, which markers should we choose? *Proj. Clin. Biol. Res.*, **269**, 43–56.

Crawford E.D., Eisenberger M.A., McLeod D.G. *et al.* (1989) A combined trial of leuprolide with and without flutamide in prostatic carcinoma. *N. Engl. J. Med.*, **321**(7), 419–424.

Denis L., Dalesio O., Murphy G. (1993) Revue de exais cliniques de phase iii sur les traitements anti-androgeniques combines (TAC) chez les patients ayant un cancer de prostate metastase. *Prog. Urol.*, **3**(1), 75–85.

De Voogt H.J., Smith P.H., Pavone-Macaluso M., de Pauw M., Sucin S. (1986) Cardiovascular side effects if diethylstilbestrol, cyproterone acetate, medroxyprogesterone acetate and estramustine phosphate are used for treatment of advanced prostatic cancer; results from European Organisation of Cancer Trials 30761 and 30762. *J. Urol.*, **135**(2), 303–307.

deWys W.D., Begg C.B., Brodovsky H., Creech R., Khandekar J. (1993) A comparative clinical trial of adriamycin and 5-fluoruracil in advanced prostatic cancer: prognostic factors and response. *The Prostate*, **4**, 1–11.

Dmochowski L., Horoszewicz J.S. (1976) Vival oncology of prostatic cancer. *Semin. Oncol.*, **3**(2), 141–150.

Eagen R.T., Hahn R.G., Myers R.P. (1976) Adriamycin (NSC-123127) versus 5-fluorouracil (NSC-19893) and cyclophosphamide (NSC-26271) in the treatment of metastatic prostate cancer. *Cancer Treatment Reports*, **60**, 115–117.

El Etreby M.F., Henderson D., Habenicht U.F., Nishind Y., Kerb U. (1986) Aromatase inhibitors and benign prostatic hyperplasia. *J. Steroid Biochem.*, **25**(5B), 867–876.

Fallon B., Olney L., Culp D. (1980) Nephrostomy in cancer patients: to do or not to do? *Br. J. Urol.*, **52**, 237–242.

Fitzpatrick P.F., Rider W.D. (1976) Half body radiotherapy of advanced cancer. *J. Can Assoc. Radio.*, **27**(2), 75–79.

Fleischmann J.D., Catalona W.J. (1985) Endocrine therapy for bladder outlet obstruction from carcinoma of the prostate. *J. Urol.*, **134**, 498.

Franks L.M. (1954) Latent carcinoma of the prostate. *J. Pathol. Bacteriol.*, **68**, 803–810.

Freiha F.S., McNeal J.E., Stamey T.A. (1989) Selection criteria for radical prostatectomy based on morphometric studies in prostate carcinoma. *NCI Monogr.*, **1**(7), 107–108.

Freyer P.J. (1920) *Clinical Lectures on Diseases of the Prostate*, 5th edition. Baillière, Tindall and Cox, London.

Gleason D.F. (1966) Classification of prostatic carcinoma. *Cancer Chemother. Rep.*, **50**, 125–128.

Greene D.R., Wheeler T.M., Egawa S. *et al.* (1991) A comparison of the morphological features of cancer arising in the transition zone and in the peripheral zone of the prostate. *J. Urol.*, **146**, 1069–1076.

Hakky S.I. (1979) Ultrastructure of the normal human urethra. *Br. J. Urol.*, **51**(4), 304–307.

Hanks G.E., Leibel S., Kramer S. (1983) The dissemination of cancer by transurethral resection of locally advanced prostatic cancer. *J. Urol.*, **129**, 309–311.

Harbitz T.B., Hangen O.A. (1972) Histology of the prostate in elderly men: a study in an autopsy series. *Acta Microbiol. Scand. Pathol.*, **80**, 756–768.

Herr H.W. (1982) Cyclophosphamide, methotrexate and 5-fluorouracil combination chemotherapy versus chloroethyl-cyclohexy-nitrosourea in the treatment of metastatic prostatic cancer. *J. Urol.*, **127**, 462–465.

Higgins C.B., Brokstein J.J., Davis F.B., Galloway D.C., Barr J.W. (1977) Therapeutic embolisation for intractable chronic bleeding. *Radiology*, **122**, 473.

Hori A., Sasada R., Matsutani E. *et al.* (1991) *Cancer Res.*, **51**, 6189–6184.

Hudson M.A., Catalona W.J. (1990) Effect of adjuvant radiation therapy on prostatic specific antigen following radical prostatectomy. *J. Urol.*, **143**, 1174.

Huggins C., Stevens R.E., Hodges C.V. (1941) Studies on prostatic cancer; effects of castration on advanced carcinoma of prostate. *J. Urol.*, **46**, 997–1006.

Huggins C., Scott W.W. (1945) Cutaneous ureterostomy with contra-lateral ureteral litagation. *J. Urol.*, **53**, 325–338.

Isaacs J.T. (1984) The timing of androgen ablation therapy and/or chemotherapy in the treatment of prostatic cancer. *Prostate*, **5**(1), 1–17.

Isurugi K., Fukutani K., Ishida H., Hosoi Y. (1980) Endocrine effects of cyproterone acetate in patients with prostatic cancer. *J. Urol.*, **123**(2), 180–183.

Iversen P., Christensen M.G., Friis E., Hornbul P. (1990) A phase ii trial of zoladex and flutamide versus orchidectomy in the treatment of patients with advanced carcinoma of the prostate. *Cancer*, **66**(Suppl. 5), 1058–1066.

Iverson P. (1994) Update of monotherapy trials with the new anti androgen, Casodex. *Eur. Urol.*, **26**, 5–9.

Kasimis B.S., Miller J.B., Kaneshiro C.A., Forbes K.A., Moran E.M., Metter G.E. (1985) Cyclophosphamide versus 5-fluorouracil, doxorubicin and mitomycin-C (FAM) in the treatment of hormone-resistant metastatic carcinoma of the prostate: a preliminary report of a randomised trial. *J. Clin. Oncol.*, **3**, 385–392.

Keen C.W. (1980) Half body radiotherapy in the management of metastatic carcinoma of the prostate. *J. Urol*, **123**, 713.

Ketering A.R., Deutsch E., Maxon H.R., Vanderheyden J.L., Libson K. (1986) The chemistry of rhenium and technetium as related to the use of isotopes of these elements in therapeutic and diagnostic nuclear medicine. *Int. J. Rad. Appl. Instrum. (B)*, **13**(4), 465–477.

Kim K.J., Li B., Winer J. *et al.* (1993) Inhibition of vascular endothelial growth factor-induced angiogenesis suppresses tumour growth in vivo. *Nature*, **362**, 841–844.

Kirk D. (1985) (Editorial) Prostatic carcinoma. *Br. Med. J.*, **209**, 875–876.

Kirk D. (1987) Trials and tribulations in prostatic cancer. *Br. J. Urol.*, **59**(5), 375–379.

Kirk D. (1993) (Editorial) How should new treatments for benign prostatic hyperplasia be arrested? *Br. Med. J.*, **306**, 1283–1284.

Labrie F., Belanger A., Kelly P.A. *et al.* (1982) Antifertility effects of luteinizing hormone-releasing hormone (LHRH) agonists. *Prog. Clin. Biol. Res.*, **74**, 273–291.

Labrie F., Dupont A., Giguere M., Borsanyi J.P., Belanger A. (1986) Advance of combination therapy in previously untreated and treated patients with advanced prostate cancer. *J. Steroid Biochem.*, **25**(5B), 877–883.

Labrie F., Lully I., Veilleux R. *et al.* (1987) New concepts of the androgen sensitivity of prostrate cancer. *Prog. Clin. Biol. Res.*, **234**(A), 145–172.

Labrie F., Dupont A., Gigiere M. *et al.* (1988) Combination therapy in both untreated and previously treated patients with advanced prostate cancer. *Prog. Clin. Biol. Res.*, **260**, 41–62.

Lancet D., Pecht I. (1975) Proceedings: A fluorescent ligand with affinity towards nitrophenyl-binding immunoglobulins. *Isr. J. Med. Sci.*, **11**(12), 1393–1394.

Leo M.E., Bilhartz D.L., Bergstralh E.J., Oesterling J.E. (1991) Prostate specific antigen in hormonally treated stage D2 prostate cancer: is it always an accurate indicator of disease status? *J. Urol.*, **145**(4), 802–806.

Lepor H., Ross A., Walsh P.C. (1982) The influence of hormonal therapy on survival of men with advanced prostatic cancer. *J. Urol.*, **128**(2), 335–340.

Loening S.A., Scott W.W., Dekernion J. *et al.* (1981) A comparison of hydroxyurea, methyl-chloroethyl-cyclohexy-nitrosurea and cyclophosphamide in patients with advanced carcinoma of the prostate. *J. Urol.*, **125**, 812–816.

Loening S.A., Beckley S., Brady M.F. *et al.* (1983) Comparison of estramustine phosphate, methotrexate and cis-platinum in patients with advanced hormone refractory prostate cancer. *J. Urol.*, **129**(5), 1001–1006.

Manni A., Santen B.J., Boucher A. *et al.* (1985) Hormone stimulation and chemotherapy in advanced prostate cancer; preliminary results of a prospective controlled clinical trial. *Anticancer Res.*, **5**(2), 161–165.

McNeal J.E., Leav I., Alroy J., Skutelsky E. (1988) Differential lectin staining of central and peripheral zones of the prostate and alterations in dysplasia. *Am. J. Clin. Path.*, **89**(1), 41–48.

McNeal J.E., Villiers A.A., Redwine E.A., Stamey T.A. (1990) Capsular penetration in prostatic cancer. Significance for natural history and treatment. *Am J. Surg. Path.*, **14**(3), 240–247.

Merrin C.E., Beckley S. (1979) Treatment of estrogen-resistant stage D carcinoma of prostate with cis diaminedichloroplatinum. *Urology*, **13**(3), 267–272.

Mettlin C., Nataranajan N., Murphy G.P. (1982) Recent patterns of care of prostate cancer patients in the US: results from the surveys of the American College of Surgeons Commission on Cancer. *Int. Adv. Surg. Oncol.*, **5**, 277–321.

Mitchell M.E., Wattman A.C., Athanasoulis C.A., Kerr W.S. Jr, Dretler S.P. (1976) Control of massive prostatic bleeding with angiographic techniques. *J. Urol.*, **115**, 692–695.

Moore M.R., Troner M.B., deSimone P., Birch R., Irwin L. (1986) Phase II evaluation of weekly cisplatin in metastatic hormone-resistant prostate cancer – a southeastern Cancer Study Group trial. *Cancer Treatment Reports*, **70**, 541–542.

Morgan W.R., Bergstralh E.J., Zincke H. (1993) Long term evaluation of radical prostatectomy as treatment for clinical stage C (T3) prostate cancer. *Urology*, **41**(2), 113–120. (Comment, *Urology*, **41**(6), 605.)

Moul J.W., Davis R., Vaccaro J.A., Sihelnik S., Belville W., McLeod D. (1989) Acute urinary retention associated with prostate carcinoma. *J. Urol.*, **141**, 1357–1377.

Moul J.W., Paulson D.F. (1991) The role of radical surgery in the management of radiation recurrent and large volume prostate cancer. *Cancer*, **68**(6), 1265–1271.

Mundy A.R. (1982) A pilot study of hydroxyurea in hormone 'escaped' metastatic carcinoma of the prostate. *Br. J. Urol.*, **54**(1), 20–25.

Murphy G.P., Natarajan N., Pontes J.E. (1982) The National Survey of Prostate Cancer for the United States by the American College of Surgeons. *J. Urol.*, **127**, 928–934.

Murphy G.P., Beckley S., Brady M.F. (1983) Treatment of newly diagnosed metastatic prostate cancer patients with chemotherapy agents in combination with hormones versus hormones alone. *Cancer*, **51**(7), 1264–1272.

Murphy G.P., Huben R.P., Priore R. (1986) Results of another trial of chemotherapy with and without hormones in patients with newly diagnosed metastatic prostatic cancer. *Urology*, **28**(1), 36–40.

Muss H.B., Howard V., Richards F. *et al.* (1981) Cyclophosphamide versus cyclophosphamide, methotrexate and 5-fluorouracil in advanced prostatic cancer – a randomised trial. *Cancer*, **47**, 1949–1953.

Nesbit R.M. (1950) Endocrine control of prostatic carcinoma; clinical and statistical survey of 1,811 cases. *JAMA*, **143**, 1317–1320.

Oesterling O.E., Rice D.C., Glenski W.J., Bergstralh E.J. (1993) Effect of cystoscopy, prostate biopsy and transurethral resection of prostate specific antigen concentration. *Urology*, **42**(3), 267–282.

Oliver R.T. (1994) Renal cell cancer; is there long term survival advantage from cytokine treatment? *Eur. J. Cancer*, **30**(A), 1214–1216.

Olson K., French T., Vallee B., Fett J. (1994) *Cancer Res.*, **54**, 4576–4579.

Parmar H., Edwards L., Phillips R.H., Allen L., Lightman S.L. (1987) Orchidectomy versus long-acting D-Trp-6-LHRH in advanced prostate cancer. *Br. J. Urol.*, **59**, 248–540.

Pavone-Macalusco M., Lund F., Mulder J.H., Smith P.H., dePauw M., Sylvester R. (1980) EORTC protocols in prostatic cancer – an interim report. *Scand. J. Urol. Nephrol.*, **55**, 163–168 (Suppl.).

Pavone-Macaluso M., De Voogt H.J., Viggiano G. *et al.* (1986) Comparison of diethylstilbestrol, cyproterone acetate and medroxyprogesterone acetate in the treatment of advanced prostatic cancer. Final analysis of a randomised phase III trial of the European Organization for Research on Treatment of Cancer Urological Group. *J. Urol.*, **136**, 624–631.

Pené F., Schlienger M., Schmitt T. *et al.* (1981) Half-body irradiation for pain relief. *Eur. J. Cancer Clin. Oncol.*, **17**, 753.

Porter A.T., Chisholm G.D. (1993) (Letter) Palliation of pain in bony metastases. *Semin. Oncol.*, **20**(Suppl. 2), 1.

Ravery V., Boccon-Gibod L.A., Dauge-Geffroy M.C. *et al.* (1994) Systematic biopsies accurately predict extracapsular extension of prostate cancer and persistent/recurrent detectable PSA after radical prostatectomy. *Urology*, **44**, 371–376.

Reed W.P., Garb J.L., Park W.C., Stark A.J., Chabot T.R., Friedmann P. (1988) Long term results and complications of preoperative radiation in the treatment of rectal cancer. *Surgery*, **103**(2), 161–167.

Rich A.R. (1935) On the frequency of occurrence of occult carcinoma of the prostate. *J. Urol.*, **33**, 215.

Robinson M.R. (1987) Complete androgen blockade: The EORTC experience comparing orchidectomy versus plus cyproterone acetate versus orchidectomy plus cyproterone acetate versus low-dose stilboestrol in the treatment of metastatic carcinoma of the prostate. *Prog. Clin. Biol. Res.*, **243**(A), 383–390.

Robinson M.R.G. (1988) Prostate cancer: early or late deferred treatment? *Clin. Oncol.*, **2**, 635–640.

Rubin P., Salazar O., Zagars G. *et al.* (1985) Systematic hemibody irradiation for overt and occult metastases. *Cancer*, **55**(Suppl. 9), 2210–2221.

Scardino P.T., Wheeler T.M. (1988) Local control of prostate cancer with radiotherapy: frequency and prognostic significance of positive results of postirradiation prostatic biopsy. *NCI Monogr.*, **7**, 95–103.

Schacher A. (1981) Wirkung von verschiedenen Verbindungen mit antiandrogener Eigenschaft auf die Wechselwirkung zwischen Hypothalamus, Hypophyse und Hoden. Thesis, Berlin.

Schellhammer P., Sharifi R., Block N. *et al.* (1995) A controlled trial of bicalutamide versus flutamide, each in combination with luteinizing hormone-releasing hormone analogue therapy, in patients with advanced prostate cancer. Casodex combination Study Group. *Urology*, **45**(5), 745–752.

Schmidt J.D., Scott W.W., Gibbons R.P. *et al.* (1979) Comparison of procarbazine, imidazole-carboxamide and cyclophosphamide in relapsing patients with advanced carcinoma of the prostate. *J. Urol.*, **121**, 185–189.

Schnall M.D. *et al.* (1991) Prostate cancer: Local staging with ERSC-MRI. *Radiology*, **178**, 797–802.

Scott W.W., Gibbons R.P., Johnson D.E. *et al.* (1976) The continued evaluation of the effects of chemotherapy in patients with advanced carcinoma of the prostate. *J. Urol.*, **116**, 211–213.

Servadio C., Mukamel I., Lurie H., Nissenuorn I. (1983) Early combined hormonal and chemotherapy for metastatic prostatic carcinoma. *Urology*, **21**(5), 493–495.

Shoskes D.A., Perrin R.G. (1989) The role of surgical management for symptomatic spinal cord compression in patients with metastic prostatic cancer. *J. Urol.*, **142**(2), 337–339.

Siddall J.K., Cooper E.H., Newling D.W., Robinson, M.R., Whelan P. (1986) An evaluation of the immunochemical measurement of prostatic specific antigen in carcinoma of the prostate. *Eur. Urol.*, **12**(2), 123–130.

Slack N.H., Wajsman Z., Mittelman A., Bruno S., Murphy G.P. (1979) Relationship of prior hormonal therapy to subsequent estramustine phosphate treatment in advanced prostatic cancer. *Urology*, **14**, 549–554.

Slevin M.L., Stubbs L., Plant H.J. *et al.* Attitudes to chemotherapy: comparing views of patients with cancer with those of doctors, nurses and the general public. *Br. Med. J.*, **300**, 1458–1600.

Smalley R.V., Bartolucci A.A., Hemstreet G., Hester M. (1981) A phase II evaluation of a 3-drug combination of cyclophosphamide, doxorubicin and 5-fluorouracil and of 5-fluorouracil in patients with advanced bladder carcinoma or stage D prostatic carcinoma. *J. Urol.*, **125**, 191–195.

Smith R.B., Walsh P.C., Goodwin W.E. (1973) Cyproterone acetate in the treatment of advanced carcinoma of the prostate. *J. Urol.*, **110**, 106

Sogani P.C., Vagaiwala M.R., Whitmore W.F. Jr. (1984) Experience with flutamide in patients with advanced prostatic cancer without prior endocrine therapy. *Cancer*, **54**(4), 744–750.

Stamey T.A., Yang N., Hay A.R., Freiha F.S., Rerwine E. (1987) Prostate specific antigen as a serum marker for adenocarcinoma of the prostate. *N. Engl. J. Med.*, **317**(15), 909–916.

Stamey T.A., Freiha F., Villers A., McNeal J. (1991) Surgical margins at radical prostatectomy. *Prog. Clin. Biol. Dis.*, **370**, 301–303.

Stamey T.A., Freiha F.S., McNeal J.E., Ledwine E.A. Whitemore A.S., Schmid H.P. (1993) Localised prostate cancer. Relationship of tumor volume to clinical significance for treatment of prostate cancer, association with metastatic levels of prostate specific antigen. *J. Urol.*, **149**(3), 510–515.

Stephens F.C. (1983) Clinical experience in the use of intra-arterial infusion chemotherapy in the treatment of cancers in the head, neck, the extremities, the breast and the stomach. *Recent Results Cancer Res.*, **86**, 122–127.

Stephens R.L., Vaughan C., Lane M. *et al.* (1984) Adriamycin and cyclophosphamide in advanced prostatic cancer. A randomized southwest Oncology Group Study. *Cancer*, **53**(3), 406–410.

Teicher B.A., Holden S.A., Gulshan A. *et al.* (1994) *Int. J. Cancer*, **57**, 1–6.

Tejada F., Eisenberger M.A., Broder L.A., Cohen M.H., Simon R. (1977) 5-Fluorouracil versus CCNU in the treatment of metastatic prostatic cancer. *Cancer Treatment Reports*, **61**, 1589–1590.

Thomas D., Balaji V., Coptcoat M., Abercrumbie G.F. (1992) Acute urinary retention secondary to carcinoma of the prostate. Is an initial channel TURP beneficial? *J. Royal Soc. Med.*, **85**, 318–319.

Torti F.M., Shortcliffe L.D., Carter S.K. *et al.* (1985) A randomised study or doxorubicin versus doxorubicin plus cisplatin in endocrine-unresponsive metastatic prostatic carcinoma. *Cancer*, **56**, 25.

Tunn U.W., Thieme H. (1982) Sepsis associated with urinary tract infection and antibiotic treatment with piperacillin. *Arch. Intern Med.*, **142**(11), 2035–2038.

Tveter K.J. (1978) Paraendocrine cancer syndrome. *Tidsskr. Nov. Large Forem*, **98**(23), 1085–1090. (English Abstract.)

Twycross R. (1993) Paradoxical pain. *Br. Med. J.*, **306** (6880), 793 (Letter); *Br. Med. J.*, **306**(6876), 473–474 (Comment).

Von Recklinghausen, F. (1891) Die Sibrose und deformiriendi Ostitis der Osteomalacie und die osteoplastichie Carcinome in ihren gegensteitizen Beziehingen. Festschr 2. *Virchow Berlin*, **1**, 89.

Whitmore W.F. Jr., Hilaris B., Grabstald H. (1972) Retropubic implantation of iodine 125 in the treatment of prostatic cancer. *Tran. Am. Assoc. Genitourin. Surg.*, **64**, 55–57.

Widmann B.P. (1934) Carcinoma of lip; results of voentgen and radium treatment. *Am J. Roentgenol.*, **32**, 211–217.

Yagoda A., Vurgrin D. (1979) Theoretical considerations in the treatment of seminoma. *Semin. Oncol.*, **6**(1), 74–81.

Yagoda A., Mukerji B., Young C. (1972) Bleomycin, an antitumor antibiotic. Clinical experience in 274 patients. *Ann. Intern. Med.*, **77**, 861–870.

Young, H.H. (1941) Fifty years progress in urology. *Am. J. Surg.*, **51**, 120.

Index

INDEX

bilateral orchidectomy combination 61, 62
cardiovascular toxicity 36
strontium, intravenous 81
strontium-89 chloride 82
surgery
  haemolytic problems 16
  management plan 23
  radical prostatectomy 51
  spinal cord compression 87, 95
survival time ix
susceptibility 9
syringe driver 92, 93

technetium salts 23
technetium-99 labelled bone scan 24–5
temazepam 94
terminal illness x, 89
testes 49
testosterone 43–4
  flair 38
  LHRH analogue effects 39
  receptor protein inhibitors 49
  removal 36, *37*
  suppression effects 39–40, 56
thermoregulation
  catecholamines 42
  disturbance 41
TNM classification 30–2
  incidental prostate cancer 31
  locally extensive cancer 31
  locally extensive tumour with
      fixation/invasion 31
  metastatic disease 32
  palpable/visible carcinoma confined within
      prostate 31
  regional lymph nodes 32
  stage grouping 32
transformation, multistep theory 8, *9*
transitional cell carcinoma 26
transrectal ultrasound (TRUS) 13, 18, 21–3,
      33, 66
  biopsy 22, 26
  false negative rate 22
  hyperechoic foci 21
  hypoechogenicity 21
transurethral coagulation 69
transurethral resection of the prostate
      (TURP) 13, 64, 69
  bladder trigone 73–4
  channel 36, 65, 67
  dissemination of cancer 65–6
  urinary retention 67
trauma, tissue 6
treatment

deferred 52, 53, 54, 63
  objective ix
trust 89
tryptorelin 38
tumour
  cell
    proliferation 6
    targeting 7
  detection marker 12
  grade
    marker 14
    PSA level 15
  progression ix, 53, 54, 56–7
  recurrence 12, 34–5
  suppressor genes
    putative genetic alterations 9
    site 10
  volume 7, *8*

ureteric obstruction 20
  bladder outflow obstruction 54, 70, *72*
  deferred treatment 54
  hormonal treatment 95
  hormone resistant disease 95
  management 70, 73
  metastatic disease 70, *71–2*, 73–4
  nephrostomy tube *72*, 73
  open urinary diversion 74
  paranodal lymphatic disease 70, *72*
  percutaneous urinary diversion 73
  post-micturition residual 70, *71*
  radiotherapy 74
  transurethral resection of bladder
      trigone 73–4
ureteric stent 73–4, 95
urethral stricture irradiation 65
urinary diversion
  open 74
  percutaneous 73
urinary retention 66–7, 69
  benign prostatic hyperplasia 67
urinary tension, acute 38

vascular endothelial growth factor 7
venereal transmission association 3
vertebral body collapse 85–8
vertebral collapse 77
vertebral crush fracture, pathological 83
vinblastine 57
vomiting 93

Zoladex 39, 47–50